The Natural Path to Wellbeing

Principles of Natural Health and Healing

Victoria Anderson

Copyright © 2025 Victoria Anderson

All Rights Reserved.

No part of this book may be reproduced, stored in a retrieval system, or transmitted in any form or by any means, electronic, mechanical, photocopying, recording, or otherwise, without the prior written permission of the publisher, except in the case of brief quotations embodied in critical articles or reviews.

Table of Contents

Introduction to Natural Healing 1
   Understanding of Natural Healing 2
   The Philosophy Behind Natural Healing 5
The Foundation of Natural Healing 9
   1. Philosophy Behind Natural Healing 10
   2. Core Principles of Natural Healing Methodology 13
   3. Core Principles of Holistic Health 17
   4. The Core Principles of Nutritional Teachings 21
   5. Understanding Foods: What to Embrace and What to Avoid 25
   6. The Role of Whole Foods and Plant-Based Ingredients in Diet 29
   7. Hydration: Understanding Its Critical Role in Health 34
   8. The Significance of Organic and Non-GMO Foods 40
   9. Combating Common Ailments with Specific Nutrients 45
   10. Implementing Nutrient-Focused Strategies 64
   11. The Importance of a Balanced pH 69
   12. Superfoods for Daily Meals 97
   13. Overcoming Digestive Disorders 111
   14. Managing Diabetes Naturally 117
   15. Heart Health and Hypertension 123
   16. Natural Solutions for Respiratory Conditions 132
   17. Addressing Skin Conditions with Herbs 138
   18. Mental Health and Stress Relief 145
   19. Enhancing Immune Function 152
   20. Women's Health: Natural Approaches 158

21.	Combating Chronic Inflammation	165
22.	Cancer Prevention and Support	172
23.	Easing Migraines and Headaches	179
24.	Natural Remedies for the Common Cold and Flu	184
25.	Men's Health: Prostate Support and Vitality	191
26.	Allergy Relief and Management	197
27.	Energizing Breakfast Recipes	204
28.	Revitalizing Lunch Recipes	211
29.	Nourishing Dinner Recipes	220
30.	Healthy Snacks and Sides	230
31.	Wholesome Desserts	239
32.	Healing Beverages	247
33.	The 30-Day Disease Prevention Routine	254

Appendix 260

Conclusion 288

Introduction to Natural Healing

Understanding of Natural Healing

Natural healing is applied through a detailed holistic approach, focusing on food consumption, lifestyle practices, and organic solutions to promote wellness and prevent illnesses. At the core of this method is the belief that the human body has self-healing capabilities that activate when provided with the right environmental conditions and essential resources. The following section outlines the methodology and fundamental principles that guide this approach.

The Core Philosophy

Achieving true health relies on maintaining a harmonious balance within the human body. Identifying the root causes of health issues is emphasized over symptom-focused medical care. This approach aims to restore the body's natural equilibrium by addressing the underlying factors that contribute to illness.

Key Principles of Natural Healing Approach

1. A holistic approach to health incorporates an analysis of physical, mental, and emotional dimensions as interconnected elements. Maintaining balance among these aspects is essential for achieving optimal well-being.

2. The fundamental principle of this medical philosophy is that food functions as medicine. A diet centered on whole, plant-based foods, particularly organic and non-GMO ingredients, is emphasized. Proper nutrition is considered essential for preventing, managing, and reversing many chronic diseases.

3. The healing process incorporates herbal medicine, natural supplements, and dietary interventions. Both traditional wisdom and

current research are used to identify suitable remedies for various health concerns, ensuring personalized solutions.

4. Health is influenced by individual lifestyle choices and environmental conditions. Essential components for healing include regular physical activity, adequate hydration, stress reduction, and living in a toxin-free environment.

5. Wellness recommendations are tailored to meet specific needs, recognizing that each person is unique. Individualized health strategies are developed through careful evaluation of medical history, lifestyle habits, and personal preferences.

Understanding of Natural Healing Methodology

An educational framework is utilized to empower individuals in taking control of their health through step-by-step guidance. This approach includes the following components:

Assessment and Education

The initial assessment involves a thorough evaluation of nutritional habits, lifestyle choices, and medical history. This process helps identify potential health imbalances or nutritional deficiencies. Education plays a central role in this approach, as informed individuals are more likely to implement lasting health improvements.

Nutritional Interventions

Clinical practices are grounded in dietary recommendations, supported by research that emphasizes a nutrition plan incorporating various food groups such as fruits, vegetables, whole grains, nuts, seeds, and legumes. A focus is placed on consuming unprocessed, sugar-free foods without artificial additives.

Herbal and Supplemental Support

Dietary modifications are complemented by carefully selected herbal remedies and supplements, chosen for their ability to support natural healing processes and address specific health concerns. Each remedy undergoes thorough assessment to ensure its effectiveness. Education on proper usage and correct dosage is provided to ensure safe and beneficial application.

Life-style Modifications

Lifestyle is considered a crucial factor in maintaining health. Daily exercise, adequate sleep, and stress reduction techniques such as meditation and yoga are emphasized. Guidance is provided on minimizing exposure to pollutants, along with strategies to improve water quality and indoor air standards.

Monitoring and Adjustment

Ongoing adjustments are essential to maintaining an effective treatment plan. Regular progress evaluations ensure that wellness strategies are modified as needed. This dynamic approach guarantees continuous effectiveness while adapting to individual health needs.

Conclusion

Natural healing care is provided through a comprehensive approach that empowers individuals to take control of their well-being through mindful choices and restorative methods. Health promotion is built on nutrition, lifestyle, and natural remedies, offering a structured framework for maintaining optimal health. Through education and support, this approach fosters long-term wellness and aids in disease prevention.

The Philosophy Behind Natural Healing

Natural healing is a wellness approach that supports the body's ability to heal itself using only natural methods. This philosophy is rooted in holistic practices, recognizing the mind, body, and spirit as an interconnected system. The key components of this approach serve as the foundation for a healthier and more balanced lifestyle.

The Essence of Natural Healing

Natural healing focuses on identifying and activating the body's innate ability to restore health. When provided with the right conditions and essential resources, the body can maintain wellness and combat illness without relying on invasive medical interventions. This preventive approach prioritizes health preservation and disease prevention over symptom-focused treatments.

Holistic Health: A Comprehensive Approach

Holistic health theory forms the foundation of this practice, treating each person as a whole being composed of physical, emotional, spiritual, and mental elements. This approach recognizes the interconnected nature of these aspects, where an imbalance in one area can affect overall well-being. Key features of holistic health in this method include:

1. A state of physical health requires balanced nutrition plus exercise and enough rest in addition to abstaining from dangerous chemicals.

2. Mental Health is promoted through stress management, positive thinking, and mental relaxation techniques.

3. The support of emotional health comes from connections between healthy people with constructive emotion expression alongside balanced emotional states.

4. Spiritual Health expands through activities such as inner self-connection together with practices of mindfulness and maintaining a clear life purpose.

Nutrition: The Cornerstone of Health

Nutrition is regarded as the primary foundation for natural healing, with wholesome food serving as a form of medicine. Unprocessed, whole foods are emphasized for their ability to provide essential nutrients needed for optimal body function. The following key nutritional principles are promoted within this approach

• A person adopting Whole Foods nutrition eats foods in their original form, including vegetables, whole grains, nuts, seeds, and fruits.

• A diet based on plants enables people to reach their nutritional needs through antioxidants, vitamins, and minerals, which come from plant sources.

• Organic and non-GMO foods are among the selection choices because they decrease chemical exposure and raise nutrient content.

• People should keep their water intake at the right levels since hydration supports both bodily operations and health.

Natural Remedies and Herbal Medicine

A combination of proper nutrition, herbal remedies, and natural treatments is emphasized to support overall health. Both traditional wisdom and modern research are utilized to identify natural healing solutions. This approach includes:

• Herbs are applied as medicinal agents to treat particular medical conditions.

• Natural Supplements that include vitamins and minerals and various other supplements help complete nutritional needs and support human bodily operations.

• Natural remedies receive proper guidance on recommended dosing practices, which ensures their safe and effective application to patients.

Life-style and Environmental Factors

Health, lifestyle, and environmental factors play a crucial role in this approach. Emphasis is placed on creating a healthy living environment and adopting behaviors that support overall well-being. Key considerations include:

• Regular exercise at appropriate levels helps people maintain their physical fitness and mental well-being.

• Two key elements combining stress management techniques, which include meditation alongside deep breathing followed by mindfulness practice for better stress control.

• Patients must protect themselves from environmental toxins by selecting natural cleaning products while remaining away from destructive chemicals and ensuring pure air and water quality.

Preventive and Personalized Care

A medical approach centered on preventive care serves as the foundation of this philosophy. By focusing on health preservation and illness prevention, the need for medical intervention is minimized. Individualized care is emphasized, tailoring health strategies to meet specific needs. This customized approach ensures long-term success and lasting benefits.

Conclusion

A holistic and preventive natural healing philosophy emphasizes the interconnectedness of all aspects of life. Supporting the body's natural healing abilities through proper nutrition, natural remedies, and healthy lifestyle choices is essential. Embracing these principles fosters health stability, empowering individuals to lead healthier and more fulfilling lives.

The Foundation of Natural Healing

1. Philosophy Behind Natural Healing

Natural healing as an approach to health recognizes that the body possesses its own healing powers, so it opts for holistic preventive treatments that support both mental and emotional well-being in addition to physical healing. The practice and teachings are built on multiple core principles that form the foundation of this philosophy.

Core Principles of Natural Healing

1. Holistic Health

Health is viewed as the integration of physical, mental, and spiritual well-being. Genuine wellness is achieved by addressing more than just physical symptoms, emphasizing the balance between emotional health, spiritual clarity, and mental wellness. These interconnected aspects influence overall well-being, where an imbalance in one area can affect the whole system.

2. Prevention Over Treatment

Preventing disease before it develops is a core principle of this approach, emphasizing proactive health management over reactive treatment. Taking control of personal well-being reduces the need for medical intervention. This program incorporates health assessments, personalized wellness plans, and educational initiatives to promote a healthier lifestyle.

3. Nutrition as Medicine

Food is promoted as a vital healing tool, with organic, unprocessed plant-based foods providing essential nutrients for optimal health. A key element of this nutritional philosophy includes:

- The strategy at Whole Foods allows customers to find unprocessed foods in their original form so they can reach their highest nutrient absorption.

- Food from plant sources remains the focus because fruits and vegetables, along with nuts, seeds, and legumes, offer an extensive measure of vitamins, nutrients, and antioxidants.

- The choice of organic produce, along with non-GMO foods, helps decrease toxic substances that the body absorbs, thereby creating less stress on the body's system.

4. **Natural Remedies and Herbal Medicine**

Herbal medicine and natural remedies are integrated into this practice, combining traditional wisdom with scientific research to select supplements that support the body's self-healing processes. This approach includes:

- Plant-derived remedies extracted from herbal sources are employed to handle particular medical problems in patients.

- The practice provides natural supplements that contain vitamins, essential nutrients, and other dietary components that are missing from regular food intake.

- All remedies, together with supplements, must follow safe usage while maintaining proper effectiveness through accurate dosage recommendations.

5. **Life-style and Environmental Factors**

Creating a supportive living environment and adopting healthy lifestyle habits are emphasized due to their direct impact on overall well-being. This includes:

- The medical staff promotes physical activity as a way to balance fitness with mental well-being.

- The practice of stress management includes teaching patients stress reduction methods such as meditation, yoga, and deep breathing for enhanced relaxation.

- Going toxin-free means people must adopt natural cleaning methods while taking care of their air quality and water purity, together with selecting harmless chemicals in their personal care products.

6. **Personalized Care**

This healthcare approach focuses on developing personalized treatment solutions tailored to individual health needs. Wellness protocols are designed based on an evaluation of medical history, personal preferences, and daily routines, ensuring a customized path to well-being. The customized method helps generate recommendations that are resilient and effective at the same time.

7. **Empowerment Through Education**

Education is regarded as a fundamental pillar of this approach, empowering individuals with the knowledge needed to take control of their own health. Providing accessible and informative guidance enables independent health management and long-term well-being. People gain better health control by studying natural healing principles to select proper wellness choices.

Conclusion

Natural healing emphasizes prevention and a comprehensive healthcare strategy, integrating nutrition, natural remedies, lifestyle adjustments, and personalized care to support the body's self-restoration. These principles guide individuals toward holistic well-being, empowering them to lead fulfilling, healthy lives. This approach focuses on disease prevention and enhances the body's natural healing abilities by recognizing its intrinsic capacity for renewal.

2. Core Principles of Natural Healing Methodology

A health approach is implemented that combines natural healthcare methods with dietary adjustments and lifestyle modifications. Essential principles focus on empowering individuals to identify the root causes of illness while supporting the body's natural healing processes. The main principles of this approach include:

1. Holistic Health Perspective

Integration of Mind, Body, and Spirit

Treatment methods take a comprehensive view of health, addressing physical, emotional, mental, and spiritual well-being. Since these aspects are interconnected, achieving true wellness requires a balanced approach. By considering the whole person, these methods and lifestyle adjustments promote optimal well-being.

2. Prevention Over Cure

Focus on Preventive Care

This approach is rooted in preventive care, emphasizing measures that maintain health and reduce the risk of disease. Regular health assessments, along with targeted lifestyle and dietary adjustments, play a key role in preventing illness and supporting overall well-being.

3. Nutrition as Medicine

Whole, Plant-Based Foods

Whole plant-based foods are considered essential for a healthy diet, with proper nutrition serving as a form of natural therapy. This approach supports disease prevention, management, and potential reversal. Key dietary principles include:

• The diet at Whole Foods consists of unprocessed plant-based and nature-fresh food that maintains essential nutrients.

• Plant-Based Diet emphasizing fruits, vegetables, whole grains, nuts, seeds, and legumes.

• Consuming organic food along with ridding sources of Genetically Modified Organisms (GMOs) helps decrease exposure to dangerous chemicals while providing better nutritional benefits to the body.

4. Use of Natural Remedies

Herbal Medicine and Supplements

Natural remedies and herbal medicine treatments are incorporated into this practice, utilizing plant-based medications and supplements to provide therapeutic support for various health concerns. This approach includes:

• Plants and their extracts are used as natural remedies to support the treatment of various health conditions.

• Natural Supplements contain vital vitamins as well as essential minerals and dietary nutrients for patients who do not receive adequate dietary nutrition.

• Natural remedies require proper safety measures along with effective realization to establish their use through appropriate dosing and blending methods.

5. Life-style Modifications

Healthy Habits and Environment

Lifestyle choices and environmental factors play a significant role in health outcomes. Emphasis is placed on creating health-supportive environments and adopting habits that enhance overall well-being. Key lifestyle modifications include:

- Regular physical activity is emphasized as a crucial factor in promoting both physical and mental well-being through consistent exercise routines.

- The program teaches stress management through meditation, yoga, and deep breathing to help patients decrease their anxiety and create relaxation states.

- People who want toxin-free living should select natural cleaning supplies for their homes and prevent exposure to dangerous chemicals through clean water, inhalable air, and safe personal care products.

6. Personalized Care

Individualized Health Plans

Healthcare is tailored to meet individual needs by considering personal health history, lifestyle choices, and preferences. This personalized approach ensures effective recommendations with long-term sustainability.

7. Education and Empowerment

Knowledge and Tools for Self-Care

Education is a fundamental component of the treatment framework, providing individuals with the knowledge and tools needed to take control of their health. Natural healing principles empower people to make informed decisions and adopt healthier lifestyles.

8.　Continuous Monitoring and Adjustment

Dynamic and Adaptive Approach

Counseling sessions focus on continuous health monitoring and adapting wellness plans to meet evolving needs. Regular assessments ensure that health strategies remain effective, allowing for necessary adjustments based on individual progress and environmental factors. This flexible approach helps optimize long-term health outcomes.

Conclusion

Comprehensive approach to health and wellness integrates multiple key elements, including holistic healing, preventive care, nutrition, natural remedies, lifestyle adjustments, personalized treatment plans, education, and regular health monitoring. By combining these principles, individuals can achieve and maintain optimal well-being, fostering a healthier and more fulfilling life.

3. Core Principles of Holistic Health

1. Integration of Mind, Body, and Spirit

Within holistic health practices, the three aspects of spirit, mind, and body unite as interconnected entities. The approach acknowledges that health problems in a single aspect will impact the entire person, while achieving wellness requires a balance between each life part of an individual.

2. Prevention and Wellness

Holistic health centers around disease prevention and maintaining complete wellness instead of providing illness treatment alone. People should actively choose healthy life habits, make well-informed nutritional choices, and develop stress management skills to avoid medical problems before they start.

3. Natural and Non-Invasive Treatments

According to holistic health philosophy, one should choose non-invasive treatments that use natural methods whenever practical possibilities arise. The healing capabilities of the body receive dual support from treatments such as herbal medicine and nutritional therapy, physical activity, and natural remedies.

4. Personalized Care

Each person requires their own personalized approach to healthcare, which forms the basis of holistic healthcare. The health care method incorporates individual health records and life choices together with personal choices and environmental conditions when creating adaptable wellness strategies that bring enduring results.

5.   **Education and Empowerment**

Education, combined with the empowerment of people, is a fundamental element in holistic health practices. The practitioners who specialize in holistic health provide their clients with knowledge combined with the necessary tools to help them achieve better lifestyle choices that create sustainable wellness.

Benefits of Holistic Health

1.   **Comprehensive Wellness**

The approach to holistic health supports wellness development through synchronization between the physical body and mental awareness, emotional health, and spiritual guidance. The complete healthcare method results in balanced health development that continues over time.

2.   **Prevention of Chronic Diseases**

The holistic health approach puts an emphasis on wellness prevention through healthy life choices to stop the formation of diabetes alongside heart disease and hypertension. People who receive timely medical interventions combined with regular maintenance of their health experience reduced probabilities of developing medical conditions.

3.   **Enhanced Mental and Emotional Well-being**

The practices of holistic health, which include mindfulness meditation and stress management, help people achieve better emotional and mental well-being. Weekly practices enable people to handle stress levels while lowering their anxiety to achieve a better quality of life.

4.   **Natural and Safe Healing**

Natural therapies combined with non-compressive treatment methods lower the probability of adverse consequences from traditional medical approaches. Safe healing practices within holistic health blend with natural body processes to create gentle treatment methods.

5. **Empowerment and Self-Awareness**

The empowerment approach of holistic health lets patients maintain complete control of their wellness development process. This increased self-awareness and responsibility for personal health lead to more informed and effective health choices.

Key Practices in Holistic Health

1. **Nutrition and Diet**

Acquiring proper nutrition serves as the fundamental principle of holistic health practice. Organic whole foods, along with healthy proportions of fruits and vegetables and whole grains along with nuts and seeds and legumes, provide bodily needs for health optimization. Medical science recognizes the importance of handling all foods that are processed along with refined sugars and artificial additions.

2. **Physical Activity**

The practice of regular physical exercise establishes primary requirements for preserving physical wellness together with adequate mental health. The combination of exercise delivers two major advantages: it benefits cardiovascular function and tones muscles while building flexibility and producing endorphin releases that boost mood.

3. **Stress Management**

The integral elements for holistic health include stress management techniques such as meditation yoga, deep breathing exercises, and mindfulness training. These mindfulness exercises serve three purposes: they minimize stress but also enhance mental concentration, and create emotional stability.

4. **Herbal Medicine and Natural Remedies**

Holistic health adopts herbal medicine and natural remedies, which serve as complementary methods to support the healing process. Herbal teas, together with tinctures and essential oils, as well as natural supplements, serve to treat particular health problems and improve complete wellness.

5.   Mind-Body Practices

The practice of mind-body techniques, which include tai chi and qigong, along with acupuncture, centers on body energy equilibrium and relaxation, which results in healing. Such health practices simultaneously protect the physical, mental, and emotional parts of the body.

6.   Environmental Health

Physical wellness demands a healthful environment at all times. People must limit their contact with environmental toxins while they should select natural cleaning products and personal care products to create a healthy environment.

Conclusion

As a whole health system, holistic health unifies physical health through its complete approach to wellness, which includes caring for mental aspects as well as emotional and spiritual elements to reach peak health. Lessons in prevention, together with personalized care, natural remedies, and educational opportunities, enable holistic health to provide people with tools to improve their overall wellness. Taxonomic health practices, including proper nutrition, physical activity, and stress management with natural remedies, enable sustained wellness to bring about total life satisfaction.

4. The Core Principles of Nutritional Teachings

Food serves as the foundation of an approach rooted in nutritional teachings. This method emphasizes whole and natural foods, which contribute to both health maintenance and disease prevention. The framework provides individuals with essential principles for using diet to support overall well-being.

1. Whole, Unprocessed Foods

Emphasis on Natural State

A diet centered on whole foods emphasizes consuming items in their natural, unprocessed state. This approach ensures the intake of essential nutrients from sources such as fruits, vegetables, whole grains, nuts, seeds, and legumes. The principle underscores the importance of the following points:

- The nutritional value of whole foods matches their density because they contain essential vitamins as well as minerals, dietary fiber, and antioxidants that promote health optimally.

- Consuming processed foods becomes harmful to health when they contain artificial ingredients because they include preservatives and refined sugars along with additives.

2. Plant-Based Diet

Rich in Plant-Based Ingredients

Plants form the core of a dietary framework that emphasizes nutrition from natural sources. This approach includes:

- An individual should eat different types of vegetables and fruits so they get diverse nutrients from each color.

- The nutritional benefits of legumes and nuts include protein, healthy fats, and fiber content, which are obtained through beans, lentils, and nuts along with seeds.

- Whole Grains provide supportive benefits to digestive health while maintaining stable blood sugar levels because people should choose quinoa brown rice and oats instead of refined grains.

3. Organic and non-GMO Foods

Prioritizing Organic Choices

Choosing organic products and non-GMO foods helps reduce exposure to pesticides, herbicides, and genetically modified organisms. The benefits include:

- Organic foods provide decreased exposure to toxins because they are grown without synthetic pesticides together with fertilizers, which decreases exposure to dangerous substances.

- The nutrient content in organic produce normally surpasses conventional farming standards to provide health benefits to consumers.

4. Balanced Macronutrients

Proper Balance of Carbohydrates, Proteins, and Fats

Maintaining the correct proportions of macronutrients supports overall bodily health by ensuring balanced energy levels, proper metabolism, and essential bodily functions. A well-structured diet include.

- Complex carbohydrates emphasize whole grains, fruits, and vegetables as primary sources of carbohydrates for sustained energy.

- The diet needs healthy fats that come from avocados, plus nuts and seeds and olive oil to help the brain and hormones function properly.

- When selecting proteins, people should focus on plant proteins and products from lean animals to enhance muscle recovery and immune system health.

5. Hydration

Importance of Adequate Hydration

Proper hydration stands as a fundamental component of a well-balanced nutritional strategy. Sufficient fluid intake plays a crucial role in supporting digestive function, maintaining circulatory health, and regulating body temperature:

- Daily consumption of water meets two essential requirements: it supports hydration and enables maintenance of bodily procedures.
- The addition of hydrating foods such as fruits and vegetables should become part of your diet because these foods have high moisture content.

6. Combating Inflammation

Anti-Inflammatory Foods

Anti-inflammatory foods serve as a key element in managing and preventing chronic inflammation, a condition linked to various health concerns. These foods include nutrient-rich options that help reduce inflammation and promote overall well-being:

- Fruits and Vegetables, particularly those rich in antioxidants, such as berries, leafy greens, and cruciferous vegetables.
- Omega-3 fatty acids are found in flaxseeds, chia seeds, walnuts, and fatty fish like salmon.
- A few anti-inflammatory foods include natural herbs like turmeric, ginger, and garlic alongside spices that control inflammation in the body.

7. Personalized Nutrition

Tailoring Diet to Individual Needs

Personalized diets are essential, taking into account factors such as age, background, physical activity levels, and specific health conditions to meet individual nutritional needs effectively:

- The first step includes a dedicated assessment process that examines dietary habits and personal health alongside life-related aspects to develop specific nutritional plans.

- Widespread evaluations and regular health status checks enable the doctor to adapt client nutritional plans according to their evolving condition.

8. Education and Empowerment

Educating for Informed Choices

Educating individuals about nutritious diets and empowering them to make informed dietary choices serves as a fundamental principle in promoting overall well-being. This involves:

- Nutritional Literacy provides knowledge about the nutritional content and health benefits of different foods.

- Practical daily recommendations help individuals adopt wellness through mindful dietary choices.

Conclusion

Nutritional guidance emphasizes whole, unprocessed foods, plant-based diets, organic and non-GMO selections, balanced macronutrients, proper hydration, inflammation control, and personalized nutrition recommendations. Educating individuals on informed food choices supports overall health and helps prevent disease through nutrition.

5. Understanding Foods: What to Embrace and What to Avoid

Foods to Embrace

Nutritional teachings emphasize two core principles: incorporating nutrient-rich foods and relying on natural, whole dietary products. These foods provide essential vitamins, minerals, antioxidants, and other beneficial nutrients that support overall health. The following information offers guidance on selecting foods to include in a daily diet.

1. Fruits and Vegetables

Variety and Color

People can find vitamins together with minerals, fiber, and antioxidants as primary components in fruits alongside vegetables. Consuming different colored fruits and vegetables produces multiple valuable nutrients in the diet. Key points include:

- Spinach, together with kale, Swiss chard, and arugula, are leafy greens that provide high amounts of vitamins A, C, K, and folate.

- Cruciferous Vegetables include broccoli together with cauliflower, Brussels sprouts, and cabbage, as these vegetables have strong cancer-fighting properties.

- Your dietary plan should include blueberries, strawberries, raspberries, and blackberries, which offer antioxidants together with fiber content.

- A combination of oranges, lemons, limes, and grapefruits constitutes an excellent addition to the daily intake because these citrus fruits contain vitamin C alongside flavonoids.

2. Whole Grains

Unrefined and Nutrient-Rich

Whole grains serve as a prime nutritional source, providing intricate carbohydrates alongside fiber and essential dietary elements. Chose whole grains including the following list:

- The protein in quinoa includes all nine essential amino acids with supplementary magnesium and abundant fiber content.

- Brown Rice provides fiber, B vitamins, and minerals like manganese and selenium.

- Oats contain beta-glucan as their main soluble fiber component, which works to decrease cholesterol levels in the body.

- Barley provides both soluble and insoluble dietary fibers that help digestion and defend against heart disease.

3. Nuts and Seeds

Healthy Fats and Protein

Seeds with nuts contain both essential vitamins and minerals along with protein fibers and healthy fats and essential proteins. Beneficial options include:

- Almonds deliver vitamin E and magnesium together with monounsaturated healthy fats reservations.

- Walnuts rich in omega-3 fatty acids, antioxidants, and anti-inflammatory compounds.

- Chia Seeds contain omega-3 fatty acids, fiber, protein, and various micronutrients.

- Flaxseeds are a good source of omega-3 fatty acids, lignans, and fiber.

4. Legumes

Protein and Fiber-Rich

Legumes serve as a superior plant-protein food that contains dietary fiber together with numerous essential nutrients. Key legumes to embrace are:

- Lentils contain high amounts of protein together with fiber and iron in addition to folate.

- White Beans supply protein with fiber together with essential folate and iron content, as well as the nutritional benefits of Chickpeas.

- Black Beans are rich in protein, fiber, and antioxidants.

- The protein content in kidney beans joins forces with fiber and multiple nutritional elements like iron and folate.

5. Healthy Fats

Essential Fatty Acids

Your body needs healthy fats because they support brain health together with hormone production as well as general wellness. The value of essential healthy fats can be found in these food sources:

- The nutritional benefits of avocados include plenty of monounsaturated fats together with fiber and potassium content.

- The healthy fats in olive oil contain monounsaturated fats alongside numerous antioxidants, thus benefiting heart wellness.

- Brands can use coconut oil because it contains medium-chain triglycerides (MCTs), which are digested easily and supply instant energy.

- Salmon and mackerel, together with sardines and trout, belong to fatty fish with their high content of omega-3 fatty acids.

6. Fermented Foods

Probiotics for Gut Health

The bacterial cultures that ferment food products bring positive health benefits to the digestive system. The essential fermented foods for consumption include:

- Yogurt provides digestive health benefits due to its alive probiotic content.

- The fermented milk product kefir combines probiotics with essential nutrients while maintaining a probiotic-rich benefit.

- Therefore, sauerkraut consists of fermented cabbage that delivers probiotics along with beneficial fiber content.

- Kimchi consists of fermented vegetables, including cabbage and radishes, that produce probiotics along with numerous vitamin contents.

Conclusion

Whole, unprocessed foods—including fruits, vegetables, whole grains, nuts, seeds, legumes, healthy fats, fermented foods, and hydrating foods—serve as essential components of nutritional health. These nutrient-rich foods support overall well-being, help prevent diseases, and align with natural healing practices and holistic wellness.

6. The Role of Whole Foods and Plant-Based Ingredients in Diet

Whole foods and plant-based ingredients form the foundation of nutritional practices that support illness prevention, overall wellness, and sustained energy levels. These essential dietary components provide vital nutrients that contribute to long-term health. The following section outlines key functions of whole and plant-based foods that should be incorporated into a daily diet.

1. Nutrient Density and Bioavailability

Rich Source of Essential Nutrients

Mosel whole food items contain vital nutrients together with fiber that enhance overall bodily health functions. The nutrients found in whole foods consistently demonstrate better bioavailability since they can be processed efficiently by the human body for useful absorption. Key benefits include:

• Warmed foods contain many important vitamins (including A, C, K, and B vitamins) and essential minerals (including magnesium, potassium, and calcium), which help various functions of the body operate properly.

• Plants contain phytonutrients that deliver three types of health benefits: antioxidants, anti-inflammatory elements, and immune system enhancers. The phytonutrient compounds include flavonoids, carotenoids, and polyphenols.

Balanced Nutrient Profile

Plant ingredients consumed intact provide a well-balanced mix of macronutrients with carbohydrates along with proteins and fats as well as micronutrients in their composition. This balance helps to:

• Because whole foods contain elaborate starches in grains and veggies, they maintain consistent energy flow in the body.

• Whole plant proteins found in legumes, nuts, and seeds function as components that repair tissues involving muscles while providing constructive growth for these muscles.

• Healthy brain function depends on the consumption of fats found in avocados along with nuts and seeds.

2. Fiber-Rich for Digestive Health

Importance of Dietary Fiber

Plenty of plant-based foods in our meals contain high dietary fiber quantities essential for good digestive system health. Fiber helps to:

• Dietary fiber produces bulk material within the stool, thereby facilitating regular bowel function and avoiding constipation.

• The soluble fiber component serves as food for beneficial gut bacteria, thus helping to develop a healthy microbiome.

• The presence of fiber in the body enables slow sugar absorption, which helps stabilize blood glucose while preventing intense fluctuations.

3. Reduced Risk of Chronic Diseases

Prevention Through Nutrition

A person who follows a dietary pattern of whole foods combined with plant-based elements has a decreased probability of developing various long-term illnesses.

- Several heart diseases become less likely when individuals eat fruits and vegetables with whole grains together with nuts and seeds, as both activities control blood pressure and cholesterol while fighting off heart disease risks.

- A plant-based diet controls blood sugar levels and enhances insulin sensitivity, which decreases the chance of type 2 diabetes occurrence.

- The preventive compounds found in plant-based foods help decrease inflammation as well as oxidative stress to protect against different kinds of cancer.

4. Anti-Inflammatory Properties

Natural Inflammation Fighters

Plant-based and whole-food ingredients exhibit anti-inflammatory substances that accomplish these effects:

- The inflammatory response weakens due to the anti-inflammatory compounds in plant-based foods, which include omega-3 fatty acids present in flaxseeds and chia seeds, as well as antioxidants within berries along with leafy greens.

- A meal plan that contains natural anti-inflammatory additives helps reduce symptoms in patients with arthritis, asthma, and inflammatory bowel disease.

5. Sustainable and Ethical Choices

Environmental and Ethical Benefits

Your health receives benefits from plant-based foods just as the environment receives benefits from whole foods, which promotes better animal welfare conditions. Benefits include:

- The environmental impact of plant-based diets remains lower than that created by animal-based eating patterns due to the requirement for minimum natural resources, including water and land.

- Your decision to cut out animal food products matches your ethical stance about protecting animals and stopping industrial farming practices.

6. Weight Management and Satiety

Supporting Healthy Weight

Your weight management can benefit from whole food consumption along with plant-based foods, which simultaneously create a feeling of satisfaction. Key aspects include:

- Whole plant-based foods have low-calorie content and abundant volume to provide satisfaction without excess food consumption.

- Eating whole foods produces satiating effects because of protein and fiber, which suppress hunger feelings, thus preventing unnecessary snacking and meal-sized food consumption.

7. Enhanced Flavor and Variety

Culinary Benefits

Different whole foods, together with plant ingredients, provide an extensive selection of taste characteristics and cooking options. Wholesome ingredients offer numerous dining possibilities that enhance your eating satisfaction. Key points include:

- The combination of fresh fruits, vegetables, herbs, and spices defines dish flavors naturally, which helps avoid the use of artificial food additives.

- Plant-based diets motivate people to investigate various food preparations while discovering diverse cultures of cuisine, which results in appreciating more satisfying eating experiences.

Conclusion

The essential role of whole foods and plant-based ingredients in dietary consumption contributes significantly to human health. These foods supply vital nutrients, promote digestive health, reduce disease risks, and offer anti-inflammatory benefits. Additionally, whole foods support sustainable and ethical eating habits while aiding weight management and enhancing flavor and variety in meals. The health advantages of incorporating whole, plant-based foods into daily nutrition align with principles of holistic wellness and natural healing.

7. Hydration: Understanding Its Critical Role in Health

Proper hydration is a fundamental element for overall well-being and optimal health. Nearly all bodily functions rely on water to support cellular health, regulate body temperature, and maintain essential physiological processes. Emphasizing the critical role of hydration promotes better health outcomes and ensures the body's systems function efficiently. This article examines different aspects of hydration and their effects on human health.

1. Essential Functions of Water in the Body

Cellular Health

Water serves as an indispensable factor for both sustaining cellular structures and allowing their proper functioning. It aids in:

- Cells achieve efficient nutrient delivery through water, which also removes waste products from the body.

- Proper hydration enables cellular communication processes to work efficiently.

Temperature Regulation

The body regulates its temperature by using water in two main processes, which include:

- When body temperature rises, sweat is created to decrease internal temperature by vaporizing perspiration.

- Adequate water levels in the body preserve blood volume, which enables correct circulation and temperature management.

Digestion and Absorption

The digestive system functions best when the human body stays hydrated. It aids in:

• The digestive system requires water to make saliva and digestive juices during the digestive process.

• Your body needs proper hydration for the intestines to absorb nutrients properly.

2. Hydration and Physical Performance

Athletic Performance

Human beings require optimal physical performance, which can only be achieved through proper hydration. Key benefits include:

• The proper functioning of muscles depends upon water because it allows muscles to contract smoothly and avoids cramp occurrences.

• The intake of water helps preserve energy levels and endurance capability in physical exercise.

Recovery

The proper hydration of the body after physical activity contributes to recovery through these three benefits:

• Fluid replacement stands essential because it restores fluid loss due to sweat activity.

• The proper hydration process enables the removal of metabolic waste products, which decrease muscle soreness.

3. Hydration and Cognitive Function

Brain Health

Your brain depends on hydrated fluids for maintaining optimal cognitive performance, which includes these abilities:

- Dehydration weakens focus and concentration abilities when it occurs.

- The proper hydration levels maintain the operation of short-term memory functions in the body.

- High water intake enables better neurotransmitter synthesis, which affects our mental condition and mood.

Preventing Cognitive Decline

Frequent periods of chronic dehydration will progressively lead to cognitive degeneration, so people must adopt excellent hydration routines from early childhood until old age.

4. Hydration and Detoxification

Kidney Function

The kidneys require sufficient water intake because only then can they perform their filtration functions properly.

- Axial and motor functions remain intact through proper water consumption, which allows the kidneys to filter waste substances from blood and produce urine.

- The right hydration level drives substances in urine away from stone formation.

Liver Function

The proper amount of water plays a vital part in helping the liver clean out waste through the following actions:

- The body requires water for metabolic processes to work properly when detoxifying.

- Proper hydration enables bile production because it serves as the basis for creating this substance, which helps eliminate waste from the body.

5. Hydration and Skin Health

Skin Appearance

The correct amount of water directly affects skin health for the following reasons:

- Body hydration helps create elastic skin that resists the formation of wrinkles.

- An appropriate water intake maintains skin moisture because it prevents dryness.

Skin Function

A proper amount of water enables the skin to operate as a protective barrier against external environmental toxins and infections.

6. Signs of Dehydration

Physical Symptoms

People must learn how to identify dehydration indicators in order to maintain their health. Common symptoms include:

- A direct indication of water deficiency in the body is thirst.

- Dry Mouth and Lips: Lack of adequate saliva production.

- Inadequate water consumption leads to dark urine that signals urine concentration.

- Dehydration leads to a major depletion of energy, and tiredness becomes very noticeable.

- A decrease in brain fluid levels results in headaches, which are one of the main physical symptoms.

Cognitive and Emotional Symptoms

Dehydration can also manifest through:

- The ability to concentrate decreases as cognitive function suffers from dehydration.
- Irritability emerges as a consequence of dehydration when it influences emotional state, which results in agitation and mental fog.

7. Recommendations for Optimal Hydration

Daily Water Intake

The recommended daily water consumption for individuals follows two general guidelines, which establish that men need 3.7 liters (13 cups) and women need 2.7 liters (9 cups) daily.

- Men: Approximately 3.7 liters (13 cups) per day.
- Women: Approximately 2.7 liters (9 cups) per day.

Factors Affecting Hydration Needs

The amount of water needed depends on various factors such as these:

- People need greater water consumption for exercise both in the middle of physical activities and after completion.
- Environmental conditions that are combined with hot and humid temperatures result in higher water loss from human sweat.
- The need for hydration depends on health conditions along with the medical treatments patients receive.

Hydrating Foods and Beverages

Hydration can be improved through drinking water as well as by consuming the following foods and beverages:

- Water-Rich Foods such as cucumbers, watermelons, oranges, and lettuce.
- Nutritious fluids include herbal teas with coconut water and fruit juice beverages.

Practical Tips

- A portable water bottle allows you to stay hydrated through small water intake periods daily.

- The implementation of alarms and reminder apps through settings helps users maintain a regular drinking schedule for water consumption.

- The goal to achieve adequate hydration and ideal urine color can be checked by evaluating its light-yellow appearance.

Conclusion

Maintaining proper hydration is crucial for overall health and well-being. Adequate fluid intake supports essential bodily functions, enhances physical performance, sharpens mental clarity, aids in detoxification, and promotes healthy skin. Establishing consistent hydration habits contributes to improved health outcomes and overall quality of life.

8. The Significance of Organic and Non-GMO Foods

Nutritional approaches emphasize organic and non-GMO foods as key elements for achieving optimal health and preventing disease. Evaluating dietary choices involves understanding the benefits of these foods and their essential role in building a well-balanced, health-supportive diet.

Understanding Organic Foods

What Are Organic Foods?

The production methods for organic foods follow systems that completely refrain from applying synthetic chemicals, including pesticides, herbicides, and fertilizers. Organic farming depends on natural processes and substances together with crop rotation, composting, and biological pest control methods.

Benefits of Organic Foods

1. Reduced Exposure to Chemicals

Organic foods reduce human contact with dangerous chemicals, which makes them attractive to consumers. The omission of synthetic pesticides and fertilizers in organic farming helps minimize health risks to people through these negative effects:

•   The endocrine system becomes disrupted when farmers apply some conventional chemicals to their crops.

•   Studies show that some pesticides generate cancer risks, which leads to carcinogenic effects in humans.

•   Continuous contact with pesticides throughout life can result in neurological issues that impact brain development.

2. Higher Nutrient Levels

Organic foods reduce human contact with dangerous chemicals, which makes them attractive to consumers. The omission of synthetic pesticides and fertilizers in organic farming helps minimize health risks to people through these negative effects:

- The endocrine system becomes disrupted when farmers apply some conventional chemicals to their crops.

- Studies show that some pesticides generate cancer risks, which leads to carcinogenic effects in humans.

- Continuous contact with pesticides throughout life can result in neurological issues that impact brain development.

3. Better Taste and Quality

Organic foods receive positive reports regarding their better sensory perception and product excellence. This can be attributed to:

- Organic farming practices build up soil fertility, which directly results in enhanced flavor and better nutritional value for harvested crops.

- Organic products contain no synthetic additives, which prevents artificial preservatives or additives from changing their taste or texture.

4. Environmental Benefits

The farming methods used in organic production combine higher sustainability and better environmental friendliness. Benefits include:

- The exclusion of synthetic chemicals supports two main environmental advantages: lowering pollution sources in both soil and water systems.

- Through organic farming, the environment earns two benefits: first, it sustains biodiversity, while second, it supports natural pest control systems with predators and preserves a variety of flora and fauna species.

- Environmental sustainability improves through crop rotation and composting, which strengthens soil structure and reduces erosion while maintaining long-term agricultural viability.

Key Organic Labels

Provide your selection of organic foods by checking for certification labels and verifying compliance with organic standards. Examples include:

- The USDA Organic label shows the product satisfies the agricultural requirements of the United States Department of Agriculture.

- EU Organic: Denotes compliance with the European Union's organic regulations.

- The certification programs for organic products operated by different nations combine to guarantee both the safety and the quality of their foods.

The Role of Non-GMO Foods

What Are GMOs?

The genetic modification process through engineered genetic techniques transforms living organisms known as Genetically Modified Organisms (GMOs). Genetic modification through genetic engineering needs genes from different species to move between species to develop valuable characteristics, including pest defense and yield enhancement.

Importance of Non-GMO Foods

1. Health Concerns

Scientists do not have complete clarity about the health risks that GMO consumption might bring in the long run. Some potential health concerns include:

- The process of adding new genes to food produces allergenic substances and raises the amount of existing allergens in food products.

- Responsible for antibiotic resistance marker deployment in GMO production, which creates the possibility of antibiotic-resistant bacterial development.

- Experimental research on GMO effects on human health continues, so medical experts warn against general GMO consumption due to possible unrecognized risks.

2. Environmental Impact

The environment experiences notable negative effects from GMO utilization that include:

- GMO plant cultivation for large areas leads to biodiversity deficiency through the displacement of native plant species and wild species. GMO resistance to herbicides creates modified crops, which demand more herbicides that produce resistant weeds alongside soil pollution.

- Repeated GMO farming operations can destroy the vitality of soil and deteriorate soil structure, ultimately harming sustainable agricultural practices in the long run.

3. Ethical and Economic Concerns

Several issues related to GMOs occur in terms of both economic and ethical aspects.

- GMO seeds undergo corporate ownership through patent systems, which restrict seed availability for farmers and cause them to remain dependent on select big companies.

- Non-GMO advocates insist that people deserve food transparency by demanding that GMOs be visibly labeled on products.

Non-GMO Certification

Check for independent non-GMO certifications on food products to determine if genetically modified organisms appear in your selected food. Examples include:

- The Non-GMO Project Verified certification program operates as a well-known GMO-free product verification standard throughout North America.

- Multiple regions, together with countries, maintain distinct labeling criteria that show products free of GMO material.

Conclusion

Organic and non-GMO foods yield various advantages to maintain optimal health through diet. Using organic foods delivers many positive health advantages through their ability to decrease exposure to dangerous chemicals while increasing nutritional values, food quality, and taste and contributing to environmental preservation. Non-GMO foods resolve several safety hazards, including medical problems and ecological challenges because of modified genes.

Selecting organic and non-GMO foods supports overall health while also benefiting the environment and encouraging mindful eating habits. This approach aligns with a holistic nutritional perspective that fosters well-being and balance through conscious food choices.

9. Combating Common Ailments with Specific Nutrients

Nutrition plays a fundamental role in maintaining overall health and preventing common health issues. The body requires specific nutrients to support various functions, including heart health, bone strength, immunity, digestion, and cognitive well-being. This section explores the essential nutrients that contribute to these key areas of health.

Nutrients for Heart Health

Heart health plays a crucial role in determining overall well-being and longevity. Certain nutrients are essential for maintaining cardiovascular function, reducing disease risk, and supporting optimal circulation. The following section explores key heart-healthy nutrients, their benefits, and the best food sources to incorporate into a balanced diet.

1. Omega-3 Fatty Acids

Importance

People need omega-3 fatty acids because they fight inflammation, normalize blood pressure levels, and reduce triglycerides while stopping blood clots from forming. These nutrients also help manage cholesterol health as they contribute to better cardiovascular wellness.

Sources

- Fatty Fish: Salmon, mackerel, sardines, trout
- Flaxseeds: Ground flaxseeds and flaxseed oil
- Chia Seeds
- Walnuts
- Algal Oil: Plant-based omega-3 supplement derived from algae

2. Fiber

Importance

Dietary fiber reduces cholesterol levels and manages blood sugar, helping people maintain a healthy weight. The digestive system uses soluble fiber as an agent to connect with cholesterol and eliminate it throughout the body.

Sources

- Whole Grains: Oats, barley, brown rice, quinoa
- Fruits: Apples, pears, berries, oranges
- Vegetables: Broccoli, carrots, Brussels sprouts, sweet potatoes
- Legumes: Beans, lentils, chickpeas, peas
- Nuts and Seeds: Almonds, chia seeds, flaxseeds

3. Potassium

Importance

The balance of sodium depends on potassium to maintain blood pressure control. Proper heart and muscle operation depends on potassium, which protects the heart from strokes and heart diseases.

Sources

- Bananas
- Oranges
- Potatoes
- Avocados
- Spinach and Other Leafy Greens
- Tomatoes

- Sweet Potatoes

4. Antioxidants

Importance

Heart protection occurs through antioxidants since they fight oxidative stress and inflammation, which separately damage blood vessels and potentially trigger heart disease. Four main antioxidants work in the body: vitamins C and E, beta-carotene, and polyphenols.

Sources

- Berries: Blueberries, strawberries, raspberries, blackberries
- Dark Chocolate: With at least 70% cocoa content
- Nuts: Almonds, walnuts
- Green Tea
- Leafy Greens: Spinach, kale, collard greens

5. Magnesium

Importance

Heart rhythm stability depends on magnesium consumption along with its ability to control blood pressure and support both muscle and nerve functioning. The human body requires magnesium to regulate essential potassium and calcium levels that are important for heart health.

Sources

- Nuts and Seeds: Almonds, cashews, pumpkin seeds, sunflower seeds
- Whole Grains: Brown rice, quinoa, whole wheat
- Legumes: Black beans, lentils, chickpeas
- Leafy Green Vegetables: Spinach, Swiss chard, kale

- Avocados

6. Coenzyme Q10 (CoQ10)

Importance

As a protective antioxidant agent, CoQ10 helps cell energy systems produce power and defends heart tissues from damage by oxidative stress. People requiring statin medications need to be especially mindful of CoQ10 depletion since these drugs lower their levels in the body.

Sources

- Fatty Fish: Salmon, mackerel, sardines
- Organ Meats: Liver, heart, kidney
- Whole Grains: Bran, wheat germ
- Nuts and Seeds: Sesame seeds, pistachios
- Spinach and Broccoli

7. Vitamin D

Importance

Heart health benefits from vitamin D because it controls blood pressure levels and minimizes inflammation while it supports entire cardiovascular functionality. The lack of vitamin D increases individuals' cardiovascular disease risk.

Sources

- Sun Exposure: The skin synthesizes vitamin D when exposed to sunlight.
- Fatty Fish: Salmon, mackerel, sardines, tuna
- Fortified Foods: Fortified milk, orange juice, cereals
- Egg Yolks

- Cheese

8. Polyphenols

Importance

Plants contain polyphenols that function as antioxidants because they decrease inflammation while enhancing endothelial function, which enables proper blood flow and heart operation.

Sources

- Berries: Blueberries, strawberries, raspberries
- Dark Chocolate: With at least 70% cocoa content
- Green Tea
- Red Wine: In moderation
- Olive Oil

Nutrients for Bone Health

People need robust bones to achieve general health status along with freedom of movement. Bone wellness relies on specific nutrients that play a crucial role in maintaining overall health. This part explains the essential nutrients needed for bone wellness and presents their advantages with corresponding food sources containing these nutrients.

1. Calcium

Importance

The human body contains the highest level of calcium as a mineral, which serves as a key component for developing and keeping robust bones and teeth together while creating powerful muscles, conducting nerve signals, and forming blood clots. The human body depends on calcium for proper muscle functioning as well as nerve communication, and prevents bleeding through clotting.

Sources

- Dairy Products: Milk, yogurt, cheese
- Fortified Plant-Based Milk: Almond milk, soy milk, rice milk
- Leafy Green Vegetables: Kale, bok choy, collard greens
- Almonds
- Tofu
- Sardines and Salmon (with bones)

2. Vitamin D

Importance

The body benefits from vitamin D through the absorption of calcium in the intestines while controlling the necessary serum levels of calcium and phosphate for proper bone mineralization. The vitamin aids both bone structure development and their recurring processes of change.

Sources

- Sun Exposure: The skin synthesizes vitamin D when exposed to sunlight.
- Fatty Fish: Salmon, mackerel, sardines, tuna
- Fortified Foods: Fortified milk, orange juice, cereals
- Egg Yolks
- Cheese

3. Vitamin K

Importance

Bone health requires vitamin K because the substance facilitates the carboxylation of osteocalcin to boost bone calcium binding and strengthen the skeletal structure.

Sources

- Leafy Green Vegetables: Kale, spinach, broccoli, Brussels sprouts
- Green Beans
- Soybeans
- Fermented Foods: Natto (fermented soybeans)

4. Magnesium

Importance

Bone formation depends on magnesium because this nutrient allows the body to turn vitamin D into its active state, which can improve calcium intake. The mineral supports the process of bone structural development.

Sources

- Nuts and Seeds: Almonds, cashews, pumpkin seeds
- Whole Grains: Brown rice, quinoa, whole wheat
- Legumes: Black beans, lentils, chickpeas
- Leafy Green Vegetables: Spinach, Swiss chard
- Avocados

5. Phosphorus

Importance

The body requires phosphorus to leverage calcium for building robust bones and teeth. Bone mineral contains this substance greatly because it maintains both bone strength and structure.

Sources

- Dairy Products: Milk, cheese, yogurt

- Meat and Poultry
- Fish: Salmon, tuna
- Nuts and Seeds: Sunflower seeds, pumpkin seeds
- Whole Grains: Oats, barley

6. Protein

Importance

The formation of new bones depends on sufficient protein because it supplies necessary building components. Proper protein consumption helps create a collagen framework for bones through its production process.

Sources

- Lean Meats: Chicken, turkey, lean beef
- Fish: Salmon, mackerel, tuna
- Legumes: Lentils, black beans, chickpeas
- Dairy Products: Milk, yogurt, cheese
- Nuts and Seeds: Almonds, chia seeds, hemp seeds

7. Vitamin C

Importance

The synthesis of collagen depends on vitamin C because collagen serves as a fundamental component of the bone matrix. Additionally, Vitamin C protects bone cells from damage caused by oxidative stress.

Sources

- Citrus Fruits: Oranges, grapefruits, lemons
- Berries: Strawberries, raspberries, blueberries

- Bell Peppers
- Broccoli
- Kiwi

Nutrients for Immune Support

1. **Vitamin C**
- **Sources:** Citrus fruits, strawberries, bell peppers, broccoli, kiwi
- **Benefits:** Boosts the production of white blood cells, enhances skin barrier function, and acts as an antioxidant.

2. **Zinc**
- **Sources:** Meat, shellfish, legumes, seeds, nuts, dairy products
- **Benefits:** Supports the immune system, aids in wound healing, and helps maintain proper growth and development.

3. **Vitamin D**
- **Sources:** Sun exposure, fatty fish, fortified foods, egg yolks
- **Benefits:** Modulates the immune response and reduces the risk of infections.

4. **Vitamin A**
- **Sources:** Carrots, sweet potatoes, spinach, kale, red bell peppers
- **Benefits:** Supports the production and function of white blood cells and maintains mucous barriers.

5. **Probiotics**
- **Sources:** Yogurt, kefir, sauerkraut, kimchi, miso
- **Benefits:** Promote a healthy gut microbiome, which is crucial for a strong immune system.

Nutrients for Digestive Health

A well-functioning digestive system is essential for overall health, as it ensures efficient nutrient absorption and effective waste elimination. Certain nutrients play a vital role in maintaining gut health by supporting digestion, reducing inflammation, and promoting beneficial gut bacteria. The following section highlights key nutrients for digestive health, their benefits, and the best food sources to include in a balanced diet.

1. Fiber

Importance

Consuming dietary fiber delivers three key benefits: Aiding in regular bowel movements, stopping constipation from occurring, and building a balanced gut microbiome. The two types of dietary fiber are soluble and insoluble.

- Solutions of soluble fiber in water create a gel-like substance that controls blood sugar and cholesterol rates.

- Insoluble fiber creates bulk in stool that helps the digestive system function through the food passage.

Sources

- Whole Grains: Oats, barley, brown rice, quinoa
- Fruits: Apples, pears, berries, oranges
- Vegetables: Broccoli, carrots, Brussels sprouts, sweet potatoes
- Legumes: Beans, lentils, chickpeas, peas
- Nuts and Seeds: Almonds, chia seeds, flaxseeds

2. Probiotics

Importance

The introduction of beneficial bacteria known as probiotics supports the optimal functioning of gut microbiology. The consumption of probiotics helps maintain healthy bacteria levels in the gut, supports digestive processes, and absorbs nutrients better while strengthening the immune system.

Sources

- Yogurt: Containing live and active cultures
- Kefir: Fermented milk drink
- Sauerkraut: Fermented cabbage
- Kimchi: Spicy fermented vegetables
- Miso: Fermented soybean paste
- Tempeh: Fermented soybeans

3. Prebiotics

Importance

Host-digestible prebiotic fibers function as dietary substances to stimulate beneficial gut bacteria, allowing them to thrive and become active. Beneficial gut bacteria use prebiotics as their nutritional base to maintain a balanced gut microenvironment and improve digestive system health.

Sources

- Garlic
- Onions
- Leeks
- Asparagus
- Bananas
- Jerusalem Artichokes
- Chicory Root

4. Water

Importance

The body needs sufficient water for digestion processes to work properly while it absorbs nutrients effectively. Water participates in nutrient dissolving, enables membrane cross-transport, and contributes to the formation of stomach acids.

Sources

- Water
- Herbal Teas
- Fruits: Watermelon, oranges, cucumbers
- Vegetables: Lettuce, celery, zucchini

5. Digestive Enzymes

Importance

Organs produce digestive enzymes that decompose food materials into easily absorbable fragments. The human body produces these enzymes naturally, and people can also derive them from particular foods.

Sources

- Pineapple: Contains bromelain
- Papaya: Contains papain
- Fermented Foods: Sauerkraut, kimchi, miso
- Raw Honey
- Avocado

6. Magnesium

Importance

The muscle contraction regulation function of magnesium assists in producing healthy bowel movements and preventing constipation.

Sources

- Nuts and Seeds: Almonds, cashews, pumpkin seeds, sunflower seeds
- Whole Grains: Brown rice, quinoa, whole wheat
- Legumes: Black beans, lentils, chickpeas
- Leafy Green Vegetables: Spinach, Swiss chard, kale
- Avocados

7. Zinc

Importance

The body maintains gut lining integrity while helping enzymes work effectively due to zinc intake, which helps strengthen the immune system.

Sources

- Meat: Beef, chicken, lamb
- Shellfish: Oysters, crab, shrimp
- Legumes: Chickpeas, lentils, beans
- Seeds: Pumpkin seeds, sesame seeds
- Nuts: Cashews, almonds

8. Glutamine

Importance

Glutamine acts as an amino acid that supports gut lining health while repairing intestinal cells and sustaining a proper intestinal barrier.

Sources

- Meat: Chicken, beef, pork
- Fish: Salmon, cod
- Dairy Products: Milk, yogurt, cheese
- Legumes: Beans, lentils, chickpeas
- Cabbage and Beets

Nutrients for Mental Health

Maintaining mental health is essential for overall well-being and quality of life. Certain nutrients play a crucial role in supporting brain function, regulating mood, and enhancing cognitive abilities. The following section explores key nutrients that promote mental health, their benefits, and the best food sources to incorporate into a balanced diet.

1. Omega-3 Fatty Acids

Importance

The brain requires two essential fatty acids, EPA and DHA, which belong to the omega-3 family, for optimal health. Brain cells depend on omega-3 fatty acids as structural elements for proper functioning, while omega-3 fatty acids also work to decrease brain inflammation and enhance brain mood and processing performance.

Sources

- Fatty Fish: Salmon, mackerel, sardines, trout

- Flaxseeds: Ground flaxseeds and flaxseed oil
- Chia Seeds
- Walnuts
- Algal Oil: Plant-based omega-3 supplement derived from algae

2. B Vitamins

Importance

The essential nutrients B6, B12, and folate benefit neurotransmission while generating energy and minimizing the chances of depression and anxiety.

Sources

- Whole Grains: Brown rice, oats, barley
- Legumes: Lentils, chickpeas, black beans
- Eggs
- Dairy Products: Milk, yogurt, cheese
- Leafy Green Vegetables: Spinach, kale, Swiss chard
- Meat and Poultry: Chicken, turkey, beef

3. Vitamin D

Importance

The molecule Vitamin D serves both functions of mood regulation and cognitive function. The lack of vitamin D creates a heightened danger of developing depression alongside other mood disorders.

Sources

- Sun Exposure: The skin synthesizes vitamin D when exposed to sunlight.

- Fatty Fish: Salmon, mackerel, sardines, tuna
- Fortified Foods: Fortified milk, orange juice, cereals
- Egg Yolks
- Cheese

4. Magnesium

Importance

The nervous system requires magnesium to control neurotransmitters and regulate stress hormone activity. The consumption of magnesium assists with controlling stress, together with anxiety and mood conditions.

Sources

- Nuts and Seeds: Almonds, cashews, pumpkin seeds, sunflower seeds
- Whole Grains: Brown rice, quinoa, whole wheat
- Legumes: Black beans, lentils, chickpeas
- Leafy Green Vegetables: Spinach, Swiss chard, kale
- Avocados

5. Antioxidants

Importance

The brain benefits from antioxidants because these substances protect the tissue from oxidative stress alongside inflammation, which impacts cognitive ability and mood. The main components of antioxidants are vitamins C and E, alongside beta-carotene and polyphenols.

Sources

- Berries: Blueberries, strawberries, raspberries, blackberries

- Dark Chocolate: With at least 70% cocoa content
- Nuts: Almonds, walnuts
- Green Tea
- Leafy Greens: Spinach, kale, collard greens

6. Zinc

Importance

Brain health, together with neurotransmitter function, requires zinc as an essential element. The inadequate state of zinc consumption leads to depression as it affects mood regulation while hindering cognitive function.

Sources

- Meat: Beef, chicken, lamb
- Shellfish: Oysters, crab, shrimp
- Legumes: Chickpeas, lentils, beans
- Seeds: Pumpkin seeds, sesame seeds
- Nuts: Cashews, almonds

7. Iron

Importance

The human body requires iron to transmit oxygen through blood, which ensures proper brain operation. A lack of iron in the body causes fatigue, together with poor concentration and mood disturbances.

Sources

- Red Meat: Beef, lamb
- Poultry: Chicken, turkey

- Fish: Salmon, tuna
- Legumes: Lentils, chickpeas, beans
- Leafy Green Vegetables: Spinach, kale
- Fortified Cereals

8. Protein and Amino Acids

Importance

Proteins contain essential amino acids that the human body needs for neurotransmitter production because these brain chemicals enable mood regulation and cognitive functionality.

Sources

- Lean Meats: Chicken, turkey, lean beef
- Fish: Salmon, mackerel, tuna
- Legumes: Lentils, black beans, chickpeas
- Dairy Products: Milk, yogurt, cheese
- Nuts and Seeds: Almonds, chia seeds, hemp seeds

9. Selenium

Importance

Selenium stands as an antioxidant substance that supports brain health functions and cognitive processes. Selenium deficiency leads to the development of mood-related disorders.

Sources

- Brazil Nuts
- Seafood: Tuna, sardines, shrimp
- Meat: Beef, chicken, turkey

- Whole Grains: Brown rice, barley
- Eggs

10. Implementing Nutrient-Focused Strategies

Consistently following a nutrient-focused approach ensures the intake of essential natural nutrients necessary for optimal health. A comprehensive nutritional method emphasizes incorporating wholesome, nutrient-dense foods into a well-balanced diet to support overall well-being. Reading this guide can give you practical instructions on how to adopt these methods in your everyday schedule.

1. Plan Balanced Meals

Key Components

• The protein group includes lean meats, fish, legumes, nuts, and seeds.

• Healthy Fats: Use sources like avocados, nuts, seeds, olive oil, and fatty fish.

• Whole Grains: Opt for whole grains such as brown rice, quinoa, oats, and whole wheat.

• Fruits and Vegetables: Fill half your plate with a variety of colorful fruits and vegetables.

Example Meal Plan

• Breakfast: Greek yogurt with berries, chia seeds, and a drizzle of honey.

• Lunch: Quinoa salad with mixed greens, cherry tomatoes, cucumbers, chickpeas, and olive oil dressing.

• Dinner: Grilled salmon with steamed broccoli, sweet potato, and a side of mixed greens.

- The recommended snacks include apple slices with almond butter as well as nuts together with hummus dips served with carrot sticks.

2. Focus on Whole, Unprocessed Foods

Benefits

- The nutritional value of whole foods exceeds that of other foods because they supply abundant vitamins and minerals together with antioxidants.

- Street cats and dogs add zero value because their diets lack artificial additives along with preservatives and extra sugars.

Tips

- Stick to shopping in the outer sections of your grocery store since you will find fresh produce as well as meats and dairy products there.

- You should prepare food at home using fresh ingredients to keep track of both quality standards and nutritional characteristics.

3. Incorporate Nutrient-Dense Snacks

Ideas

- The mixture of dried fruits with various nuts without added sugar constitutes a nutritious option.

- Normalizing healthy snacking involves presenting veggie sticks with hummus dip through ready-cut combinations of bell peppers, celery, and carrot sticks.

- Smoothies: Blend fruits, leafy greens, a source of protein (like Greek yogurt or protein powder), and a healthy fat (like avocado or nut butter).

4. Stay Hydrated

Importance

•   Drinking water is crucial for digestion alongside nutrient absorption, and it enables proper functioning of all bodily processes.

Strategies

•   Drinking at least two liters of water distributed into eight cups per day represents an optimal goal since you should modify your intake depending on your physical activities and environmental temperatures.

•   Among water-rich foods, we should eat cucumbers, watermelon, oranges, and lettuce.

5. Optimize Nutrient Absorption

Tips

•   The absorption of nutrients becomes better when pairing different foods, such as vitamin C-rich foods, with iron-rich foods.

•   Foods containing healthy fats should accompany meals because they help your body properly absorb vitamins A, D, E, and K.

•   The consumption of antinutrients needs to be reduced through soaking, followed by fermentation of grains and legumes.

6. Monitor Portion Sizes and Variety

Balance and Moderation

•   Pay attention to the sizes of your portions, as excessive eating remains possible regardless of using healthy components.

•   A diverse diet that incorporates all necessary nutrients should be maintained.

Tools

- Plate Method: Fill half your plate with vegetables and fruits, one-quarter with protein, and one-quarter with whole grains.

- Isolating food first helps people regulate their food amounts and create healthy eating plans for each meal.

7. Supplement Wisely

When Necessary

- Assessment: Identify potential nutrient deficiencies through dietary assessment and consultation with a healthcare professional.

- High-quality supplements should be selected when filling nutritional gaps becomes necessary.

Common Supplements

- High-quality multivitamins act as a solution for average nutritional deficiencies.

- Vitamin D: Especially in regions with limited sunlight.

- The recommended supplement for people with low levels of Omega-3 Fatty Acids is fish oil capsules.

8. Practice Mindful Eating

Benefits

- Your awareness of hunger and fullness signals leads to avoiding overeating because of better understanding.

- Enjoyment: Enhances the enjoyment of food and the eating experience.

Techniques

- Chew each bite slowly until you thoroughly digest your food while enjoying it thoroughly.

- People should eat without distractions from TV or smartphones since these devices take away focus from the meal.

9. Regularly Review and Adjust Your Diet

Stay Adaptable

- People should modify their dietary techniques to meet changing healthcare requirements, lifestyle patterns, and nutritional requirements.

- You should listen to your body signs and obtain medical expert feedback about your diet.

Regular Check-Ins

- Annual evaluations of nutritional values need to match health objectives while adopting a monthly review process for dietary analysis.

Conclusion

To achieve nutrient-focused nutrition, you must design well-balanced food meals that use whole foods while including nutrient-rich snacks and drinking adequate fluids alongside optimal digestive absorption and right portion control along with wise supplementation, mindful food consumption, and consistent diet evaluation. These applied steps guide you to obtain the necessary essential nutrients required for maximum health according to natural nutrition and wellness approach.

11. The Importance of a Balanced pH

The human body needs proper pH balance to support health as well as well-being at all times. Maintaining a balanced intake of alkaline and acidic foods supports optimal body function and overall well-being. The following guide examines how pH balance matters in combination with explanations about alkaline versus acidic foods while offering useful methods to establish a pH-neutral diet.

Understanding Body pH and Health

What is pH?

The measurement of substance acidity or alkalinity extends from zero to fourteen using the pH scale. A neutral substance measures 7 on a pH scale, but acidic substances have lower numbers below 7, and alkaline mixtures have higher numbers above 7. A slightly alkaline pH level of 7.4 establishes itself as the normal state of the human body because it enables essential physiological activities.

Importance of pH Balance

Maintaining a balanced pH is vital for:

•   Several enzymes in the body require particular pH conditions to execute their biochemical reaction functions properly.

•   The efficient absorption of nutrients in the digestive tract occurs through proper pH balance.

•   Body detoxification paired with waste removal becomes more effective when pH levels are at their proper levels.

•   An acidic environment affects bone density since it decreases the removal of bone minerals such as calcium after preventing such conditions.

Alkaline vs. Acidic Foods

Alkaline Foods

The body achieves its proper pH balance when we consume alkaline foods since these substances neutralize bodily acids. Such food items deliver high amounts of vitamins along with minerals and antioxidants.

Common Alkaline Foods

•	Fruits: Citrus fruits (lemons, limes), melons, berries, apples, pears, grapes, mangoes

•	Vegetables: Leafy greens (spinach, kale), cucumbers, broccoli, cauliflower, bell peppers, carrots, celery

•	Nuts and Seeds: Almonds, chia seeds, flaxseeds

•	Legumes: Lentils, chickpeas, green beans

•	Herbs and Spices: Ginger, garlic, turmeric, basil, parsley

Acidic Foods

Eating large amounts of acidic meals will make the body become more acidic. You should blend acidic foods with alkaline ones to achieve proper balance.

Common Acidic Foods

•	Animal Proteins consist of meat alongside poultry, and fish and eggs serve as such proteins, too.

•	Dairy Products: Cheese, milk, yogurt

•	Grains: Wheat, rice, oats, corn

•	Processed Foods with artificial sweeteners and refined grains, fast food, sugary snacks, and sugary foods make up the category.

•	Drinking coffee and alcohol while consuming soda and energy beverages results in increased body acid levels.

The Potential Benefits of an Alkaline Diet

Reducing Chronic Disease Risk

Alkaline diets appear to decrease the occurrence of chronic diseases through these benefits:

- Alkaline foods contain anti-inflammatory properties that work to decrease the chronic inflammatory response, which affects numerous diseases.

- An alkaline diet reduces bone mineral loss because it lets the body minimize the process of extracting minerals from bones as part of acid neutralization, therefore promoting stronger bone structures.

- Stimulating kidney operation improves through decreased dietary acid content because it reduces kidney stress, which helps prevent kidney stones.

Boosting Energy Levels

A health-balanced pH serves to enhance energy resources by:

- Shower cellular functionality operates efficiently because proper pH maintains cellular energy production abilities.

- The metabolism benefits from alkaline food, which helps minimize the effects of fatigue.

Supporting Digestive Health

Taking in alkaline substances benefits the digestive system through the following outcomes:

- Gut Flora stays in balance when you consume alkaline foods because these foods help develop healthy gut bacteria that improve digestion and nutrient absorption.

- The consumption of less acidic foods helps stop acid reflux and its associated digestive disturbances.

Implementing a pH-Balanced Diet

Practical Steps

1. Consumers should eat more alkaline fruits and vegetables, nuts, seeds, and legumes to achieve a balanced diet.

2. People should reduce their consumption of meat products, dairy products, and processed foods together with sugary beverages.

3. Drinking hydration promotes pH balance maintenance and supports detoxification through its process.

4. Eat food combinations that unite alkaline ingredients with acidic items while maintaining a well-balanced division between them.

5. Add herb and spice combinations to prepare meals that keep your body environment alkaline.

Sample Meal Plan

- Breakfast: Smoothie with spinach, kale, banana, berries, chia seeds, and almond milk.

- Lunch: Quinoa salad with mixed greens, cherry tomatoes, cucumbers, chickpeas, and olive oil-lemon dressing.

- Dinner: Grilled salmon with steamed broccoli, sweet potatoes, and a side of mixed greens.

- The recommended snacks consist of slices of apples served with almond butter and carrot sticks accompanied by hummus and a portion of nuts.

Considerations and Balance

Individual Needs

The implementation of a pH-balanced diet requires a specific evaluation of individual health conditions together with diet requirements. One can get specific nutritional advice through discussions with healthcare professionals along with nutritionists.

Avoid Extremes

The benefits of eating alkaline foods remain true, yet a person must preserve dietary equilibrium. Individual health suffers when people follow strict dietary limits because such restrictions cause both nutritional deficiencies and medical complications.

Conclusion

Pursuing a diet consisting of alkaline-rich foods enables proper pH regulation while helping people prevent disease conditions and boosting their energy levels and digestive capabilities. A healthier overall pH balance emerges when you feed your body with adequate amounts of fruits, vegetables, nuts, seeds, and legumes and control acidic food intake simultaneously. This approach aligns with holistic standards of nutrition and well-being, promoting a healthy, active lifestyle.

Understanding Body pH and Health

A properly balanced body pH stands as an essential requirement to achieve both health excellence and life well-being. Body pH serves as an important factor that controls several body functions and affects total health status. This guide examines both body pH functioning and its importance in health and provides functional methods for pH maintenance.

What is pH?

The acidity level or alkalinity of anything falls under the measurement method known as pH, which ranges between 0 to 14.

- pH 7: Neutral

- pH < 7: Acidic

- pH > 7: Alkaline (or basic)

Body pH Levels

Each body area maintains unique pH values that match its purpose:

- Blood: Slightly alkaline, with a pH around 7.35-7.45.

- The stomach environment ranges between 1.5 and 3.5 pH because its acidic nature helps the digestive process.

- The pH value of urine ranges from acidic to alkaline, between 4.5 and 8, depending on diet intake, hydration levels, and metabolic processes.

Importance of pH Balance

Enzyme Function

Numerous biochemical reactions in the body heavily depend on enzymes whose optimal operation requires specific pH ranges. The metabolic processes become disrupted when enzyme activity is affected because of pH imbalances.

Nutrient Absorption

The proper chemical balance of pH within the stomach and intestinal regions enables the body to effectively break down nutrients and absorb them into the bloodstream. For example:

- An acidic stomach environment enables efficient food processing through mineral absorption of calcium, magnesium, and zinc.

- The digestive enzyme performance in the intestinal tract demands this specific alkalinization level for maximum functionality.

Detoxification

The detoxification activities of the body mostly occur in the liver and kidneys, which need appropriate pH levels to function effectively. The pH balance enables these organs to efficiently deactivate harmful toxins.

Bone Health

The prolonged existence of an acidic body environment known as acidosis causes bones to lose minerals to reduce acidity, thus leading to weak bones and elevating the risk of osteoporosis.

Immune Function

The body requires an optimal pH level for its immune system to function at its peak capacity. Excessive acid levels in the body decrease immune response strength and create vulnerability to diseases as well as infections.

Factors Affecting Body pH

Diet

The pH balance pattern of the body depends heavily on the kinds of food and drink people consume. Food consumption affects body pH because eating acidic items will reduce pH values while eating alkaline items raises them.

Hydration

Good hydration maintains the optimal pH levels of blood and urine, which helps improve overall metabolic processes and detoxification.

Stress

Excessive stress produces more body acids, which may alter pH levels and negatively affect health performance.

Physical Activity

Physically active people enjoy better pH balance because their circulation system functions optimally while delivering nutrients more efficiently and removing wastes promptly.

Strategies to Maintain a Balanced pH

Diet

1. The addition of acidic foods like fruits, vegetables, nuts, seeds, and legumes should be encouraged in every diet.

   Examples: Spinach, kale, cucumbers, broccoli, apples, berries, almonds, and lentils.

2.   People should minimize their consumption of meat products, dairy items, processed foods, and sugar-filled beverages.

Examples: Red meat, cheese, white bread, soda, and alcohol.

3.   The proper combination of acidic and alkaline foods makes up a balanced eating pattern.

A piece of grilled chicken (acidic) can be properly balanced when served together with a large salad (alkaline).

Hydration

•   The daily goal for water consumption should be eight cups (2 liters), but you should adjust your water intake to fit your level of physical activity and climate conditions.

•   Herbal teas help hydration while supplying beneficial nutrients through their consumption.

Stress Management

•   Regular practice of relaxing techniques includes meditation and yoga, deep breathing exercises, and mindfulness in your daily activities.

•   Regular physical exercises help control stress while maintaining overall health, so practice them frequently.

Monitoring pH Levels

•   Regular urine pH surveillance happens through pH test strip monitoring. The use of pH test strips enables you to measure the levels of acid and alkaline in your body.

•   Follow up on dietary changes after measuring pH to support optimal balance.

Conclusion

A body should sustain an appropriate pH value to achieve health standards and wellness measures. A body with a balanced pH enables all essential body functions, including enzyme function, nutrient absorption, detoxification, bone health, and immune function. Your acid-alkaline body balance benefits from eating alkaline-rich foods together with hydration practices, stress reduction, and pH level tracking methods. The health and disease prevention strategies support the principles of holistic wellness because they work toward the betterment of complete health.

Alkaline vs. Acidic Foods

Understanding the differences between alkaline and acidic foods is crucial for maintaining a balanced body pH. Incorporating more alkaline foods into daily meals supports overall health and well-being. The guide provides details about alkaline and acidic food features along with their physiological effects while teaching presentable tips for diet equilibrium.

Alkaline Foods

Characteristics

The consumption of alkaline foods helps control body acid levels by balancing pH values and reducing acid build-up. The vitamins, together with minerals and antioxidants, are abundant in these foods.

Benefits

- The consumption of alkaline foods decreases body inflammation.

- Your dietary consumption of alkaline foods blocks acid accumulation in your body, which helps protect your bone structure and prevents osteoporosis development.

- A neutral pH value enables the immune system to work at its peak effectiveness.

- The consumption of alkaline foods creates a favorable condition in the digestive system to support digestive health.

Common Alkaline Foods

Fruits

- Citrus Fruits: Lemons, limes, oranges
- Berries: Strawberries, blueberries, raspberries
- Melons: Watermelon, cantaloupe, honeydew
- Other Fruits: Apples, pears, grapes, mangoes

Vegetables

- Leafy Greens: Spinach, kale, Swiss chard, arugula
- Cruciferous Vegetables: Broccoli, cauliflower, Brussels sprouts, cabbage
- Root Vegetables: Carrots, beets, radishes, sweet potatoes
- Other Vegetables: Cucumbers, celery, bell peppers, zucchini

Nuts and Seeds

- Almonds
- Chia Seeds
- Flaxseeds
- Pumpkin Seeds

Legumes

- Lentils
- Chickpeas
- Green Beans

Herbs and Spices

- Ginger
- Garlic

- Turmeric
- Basil
- Parsley

Acidic Foods

Characteristics

Acidic foods can lower the body's pH if consumed in excess. While some acidic foods are necessary for a balanced diet, overconsumption can lead to health issues.

Potential Health Issues

- The body can experience increased inflammatory responses because of eating too many acidic foods.

- Wooden bones become less dense due to the mineral leaching that happens when acid levels become too high.

- Extremely acidic diets will lead to digestive issues that disrupt gut microbiome balance and cause digestive health problems.

- High levels of acid create a negative effect on the immune system through reduced efficiency.

Common Acidic Foods

Animal Proteins

- Red Meat: Beef, pork, lamb
- Poultry: Chicken, turkey
- Fish: Tuna, salmon, mackerel
- Eggs

Dairy Products

- Cheese

- Milk
- Yogurt

Grains

- Wheat: Bread, pasta, pastries
- Rice
- Oats
- Corn

Processed Foods

- Sugary Snacks: Candy, cookies, cakes
- Refined Grains: White bread, white rice
- Fast Food: Burgers, fries, pizza
- Artificial Sweeteners: Aspartame, saccharin

Beverages

- Coffee
- Alcohol
- Soda
- Energy Drinks

Practical Tips for Balancing Your Diet

Increase Alkaline Foods

1. Make foods from the fruit and vegetable category the main portion of each meal by selecting various vibrant produce options.

2. You should eat nuts and seeds as snacks with salads and yogurt since they contain almonds and flaxseeds along with chia seeds.

3. As a protein source for meals, choose a combination of lentils, chickpeas, and different types of beans.

4. The use of alkaline herbs and spices such as ginger, garlic, and parsley should flavor your meals.

Moderate Acidic Foods

1. Limit your consumption of sugary snacks and refined grains together with fast food.

2. Select lean proteins from fish along with lean meats while providing yourself with abundant vegetables.

3. Eat dairy products carefully with small portions while substituting dairy items with plant-derived choices.

4. Refrain from consuming alcoholic sugary beverages along with coffee in moderation. Selecting water and herbal teas, along with creating green smoothies, forms a healthy choice.

Balanced Meals

1. You should include both alkaline and acidic components in each meal because this creates a mealtime balance. The recommended meal includes acidic grilled chicken together with alkaline mixed greens and cucumbers with bell peppers along with neutral quinoa.

2. The consumption of water should be substantial to facilitate toxin elimination as well as pH equilibrium maintenance.

Sample Daily Meal Plan

- Breakfast: Smoothie with spinach, kale, banana, berries, chia seeds, and almond milk.
- Lunch: Quinoa salad with mixed greens, cherry tomatoes, cucumbers, chickpeas, and olive oil-lemon dressing.
- Dinner: Grilled salmon with steamed broccoli, sweet potatoes, and a side of mixed greens.

•   You should consume apple slices paired with almond butter while carrots are dipped in hummus and a little bit of nuts.

Conclusion

The identification of alkaline and acidic foods, along with their effects on pH levels in your body, constitutes essential knowledge for maintaining proper health. Your body will achieve better pH balance when you consume alkaline foods together with limiting acidic foods, which simultaneously reduces inflammation and supports bone health. Dietary recommendations focused on holistic nutrition promote sustainable health and vitality by emphasizing whole, natural foods and balanced eating habits.

The Potential Benefits of an Alkaline Diet

An alkaline diet is suggested for its potential benefits in balancing body acidity, reducing inflammation, strengthening bones and kidneys, and enhancing daily energy levels. The following guideline examines the health advantages of alkaline eating while also offering specific daily advice for its implementation.

The Main Advantages of Following an Alkaline Dietary Plan

1.   Reducing Chronic Inflammation

Benefits

•   When consumed regularly, alkaline foods provide two main advantages: they contain antioxidants and phytonutrients that fight against body inflammation.

•   The relationship between chronic inflammation and these diseases results in an elevated disease risk, which includes heart disease together with diabetes and certain forms of cancer. When inflammation decreases, it becomes possible to decrease your odds of developing such health conditions.

Alkaline Foods to Include

- Leafy Greens: Spinach, kale, Swiss chard
- Fruits: Berries, citrus fruits, melons
- Nuts and Seeds: Almonds, chia seeds, flaxseeds
- Herbs and Spices: Turmeric, ginger, garlic

2. Improving Bone Health

Benefits

The body preserves valuable minerals through the alkaline diet since it stops essential minerals such as calcium from leaving bones to protect bone density and strength.

The support that an alkaline diet provides to bone health results in lowered osteoporosis risks together with associated fracture risks.

Alkaline Foods to Include

- Vegetables: Broccoli, cauliflower, Brussels sprouts
- Legumes: Lentils, chickpeas, green beans
- Nuts and Seeds: Almonds, pumpkin seeds
- Fruits: Apples, pears, grapes

3. Enhancing Kidney Function

Benefits

Reduction of dietary acid levels through proper nutrition helps eliminate strains from kidneys, improve organ performance, and minimize kidney stone formation.

The kidneys benefit from the alkaline diet by using its support to remove toxins and waste effectively from the human body.

Alkaline Foods to Include

- Hydrating Foods: Cucumbers, watermelon, oranges
- Vegetables: Celery, zucchini, leafy greens
- Fruits: Melons, berries, citrus fruits
- Herbal Teas: Chamomile, peppermint, ginger tea

4. Boosting Energy Levels

Benefits

A balanced pH helps cells execute their biological processes while producing energy optimally.

The alkaline diet works to decrease exhaustion levels due to its ability to maximize body performance while reducing metabolic acid carga.

Alkaline Foods to Include

- Whole Foods: Fresh fruits and vegetables, nuts, seeds
- Smoothies: Made with leafy greens, berries, and almond milk

The recommended snacks consist of apple slices paired with almond butter, while carrot sticks are consumed with hummus as a dip.

5. Supporting Digestive Health

Benefits

Healthy gut flora development occurs due to alkaline foods that support gastrointestinal health and nutritional absorption.

Acid Reflux symptoms decrease because a reduction in food acidity helps protect against reflux occurrences.

Alkaline Foods to Include

- Fermented Foods: Sauerkraut, kimchi, kefir
- Vegetables: Broccoli, carrots, celery

- Fruits: Berries, melons, apples
- Herbs and Spices: Basil, parsley, ginger

Practical Tips for Incorporating an Alkaline Diet

1. Increase Alkaline Foods

Daily Recommendations

- Your daily meals should contain half of your plate dedicated to various colorful fruits and vegetables.

- The daily diet should include one small serving of nuts and seeds to use as snacks or decorations for salads and yogurt.

- Legumes: Use lentils, chickpeas, and beans as protein sources in meals.

2. Moderate Acidic Foods

Daily Recommendations

- Stick to unprocessed foods since you should minimize sugar snacks together with refined grains and fast food consumption.

- Avoid red or processed meats, but consume lean fish and combine these proteins with vegetable portions that extend beyond half of your plate.

- People should restrict their intake of either coffee or alcoholic beverages or drinks with sugar content. Drink primarily water and herbal teas as well as green smoothies instead of other drinks.

3. Balanced Meals

Daily Recommendations

- Each meal should include both alkaline and acidic foods to establish mealtime balance according to the daily recommendations. The example meal includes grilled chicken served with large amounts of mixed greens alongside cucumbers and bell peppers together with quinoa as a side.

4. **Stay Hydrated**

Daily Recommendations

• People need to drink at least 8 cups of water (2 liters each day), yet they must modify this amount according to their activity levels and environmental conditions.

• Consuming hydrating foods like cucumbers along with watermelon, oranges, and lettuce should be included in your diet.

5. **Regular Monitoring**

Daily Recommendations

• Urine pH Test with pH test strips provides daily monitoring of acid-alkaline body balance through urine tests.

• Monitor diet by following pH reading results in order to preserve normal balance in your system.

Conclusion

The consumption of alkaline foods delivers multiple health advantages because they minimize ongoing inflammation and strengthen bones. It also helps kidney function, increases vitality, and benefits gut health. Your overall health benefits when you increase your alkaline food consumption while limiting acidic foods because this action creates a pH balance in your body. A holistic nutritional approach aligns with recommendations for an alkaline diet, promoting long-term health and vitality.

Implementing a pH-Balanced Diet

A pH-balanced eating plan requires you to add foods that support your body, achieving light alkalinity in its pH levels. Such a dietary approach enhances body health, decreases inflammation, and improves metabolic performance. The following advice and concrete steps will help you successfully follow a pH-balanced eating plan.

1. **Increase Alkaline Foods**

Fruits

Consumers should include various alkalizing fruits in their food choices.

• The body maintains alkalinity through citrus fruits, where lemon, lime, and orange serve as examples despite their acidity.

• Berries: Strawberries, blueberries, raspberries

• Melons: Watermelon, cantaloupe, honeydew

• Other Fruits: Apples, pears, grapes, mangoes, bananas

Vegetables

Choose various vegetable options that promote body alkalinity for your meals.

• Leafy Greens: Spinach, kale, Swiss chard, arugula

• Cruciferous Vegetables: Broccoli, cauliflower, Brussels sprouts, cabbage

• Root vegetables such as carrots, beets, radishes, and sweet potatoes should also be included.

• Other Vegetables: Cucumbers, celery, bell peppers, zucchini

Nuts and Seeds

Use these foods as they bring alkalizing properties when you eat them:

• Almonds

• Chia Seeds

• Flaxseeds

• Pumpkin Seeds Legumes

Legumes

Use legumes as a source of protein and fiber:

- Lentils
- Chickpeas
- Green Beans, Herbs and Spices

Herbs and Spices

Enhance flavor and alkalinity with herbs and spices:

- Ginger
- Garlic
- Turmeric
- Basil
- Parsley

2. **Moderate Acidic Foods**

Animal Proteins

Eating dietary fats is essential for dietary balance yet food consumption should be measured for maximum effectiveness.

- There are two rules for red meat that people should follow: first limit its consumption but choose only lean portions.
- Poultry: Opt for chicken and turkey
- The recommended fish for consumption include salmon, mackerel along with sardines.
- Eggs should be consumed moderately through the consumption of premium-quality eggs.

Dairy Products

Food choices should include dairy products in small amounts:

- Cheese
- Milk
- Yogurt

Grains

Balance your intake of grains:

- Wheat: Bread, pasta, pastries
- Rice
- Oats
- Corn

Processed Foods

People must reduce their intake of processed foods together with foods high in sugar:

- Sugary Snacks: Candy, cookies, cakes
- Refined Grains: White bread, white rice
- Fast Food: Burgers, fries, pizza
- Artificial Sweeteners: Aspartame, saccharin

Beverages

Monitor your drink choices carefully

- Have only two small coffee servings per day
- Alcohol: Drink in moderation
- Soda: Avoid sugary and diet sodas
- Energy Drinks: Limit or avoid

3. **Balanced Meals**

Combining Foods

Spread your meals between alkaline and acidic foods at every meal.

- Example Breakfast: Smoothie with spinach, kale, banana, berries, chia seeds, and almond milk.

- Example Lunch: Quinoa salad with mixed greens, cherry tomatoes, cucumbers, chickpeas, and olive oil-lemon dressing.

- Example Dinner: Grilled salmon with steamed broccoli, sweet potatoes, and a side of mixed greens.

- Healthy Snacks for the Day Include Peanut Butter with Apples and Carrots Served with Hummus Plus a Small Serving of Nuts.

Meal Planning

You should develop balanced meals ahead of time because this approach helps you maintain a steady intake of alkaline foods:

- Make ready portions of your food ahead of time so your meals contain multiple alkaline foods.

- Similar to other healthy foods, avoid overeating by carefully managing your food portions.

4. **Stay Hydrated**

Water Intake

The consumption of adequate water helps regulate pH levels in the body:

- The daily water consumption should be set at a minimum of 2 liters, which can be adjusted according to physical movement and environmental conditions.

- The diet should contain hydrating foods, including cucumbers together with watermelon, oranges, and lettuce, because of their high-water content.

Herbal Teas

Beneficial nutrients accompany hydration when you choose herbal teas as your source of fluid.

- Examples: Chamomile, peppermint, ginger tea

5. Monitor and Adjust

Regular Monitoring

Begin a routine practice of checking your body's pH balance through regular measurements.

- The urine pH level can be checked through the use of pH test strips to determine the solution acidity.

- Use results from pH testing to modify your dietary plan in order to reach optimal balance.

Feedback and Adaptation

Your body provides feedback signals, which you should use to modify your approach as required.

- Health Changes require the modification of dietary approaches related to adjustments in health status or lifestyle and nutritional requirements.

- Seek professional medical advice to get assistance in determining proper dietary food choices.

6. Practice Mindful Eating

Eating Habits

Creating mindful eating practices serves as a valuable approach to maintaining pH balance through diet.

- Thorough chewing should take place during each meal while enjoying each bite slowly.

- Minimal distractions should be present during meals since television and smartphones affect focus on your food.

Portion Control

Pay attention to serving sizes to prevent excessive consumption of food:

- Plate Method: Fill half your plate with vegetables and fruits, one-quarter with protein, and one-quarter with whole grains.

Conclusion

Integration of pH-balanced nutrition includes high consumption of alkaline foods while regulating acid-forming foods and keeping yourself properly hydrated, together with pH measurement and reflective eating habits. Following this method helps users achieve pH stability, which supports health goals and minimizes the threat of long-term health conditions. pH-balanced nutrition supports holistic dietary practices, contributing to long-term health benefits.

Considerations and Balance in Implementing a Balanced Diet

Your success in pH-balanced diet implementation depends on considering everything carefully while maintaining appropriate nutritional balance to prevent health problems. People should use nutrition to create balance while making controlled diet decisions. The guide outlines essential principles together with portability methods to balance the execution of a pH-balanced diet.

Key Considerations

Individual Nutritional Needs

Personalized Approach

- Health Conditions: Consider any existing health conditions. People who have diabetes along with kidney disease and osteoporosis must modify their diet according to their medical requirements.

- The nutritional demands of people change because of their age combined with gender identity and their current life cycle stage, which includes pregnancy or menopause.

- Active individuals need to eat a diet in proportion to their activity intensity because it determines their energy and nutrient needs.

Professional Guidance

- A Nutritionist should guide you regarding your diet to establish eating habits that support your unique health requirements.

- Regular medical appointments let you track your nutritional health status and require proper changes when needed.

Nutrient Balance

Avoiding Extremes

- The diet plan needs moderation because consuming only alkaline foods could lead to nutritional deficiencies.

- You must maintain a balanced diet with carbohydrates, proteins, fats, vitamins, and mineral elements.

Food Variety

- A complete dietary plan requires you to consume various types of fruits, vegetables, grains, and proteins, as well as incorporate fats to get complete nutrient coverage.

- The use of colorful plates in your meals is essential because distinct meal colors indicate different nutritional values and antioxidant content.

Food Quality

Organic and Non-GMO Foods

- People who want to minimize their pesticide exposure should select organic produce from their food options.

- You can secure non-GMO ingredients by purchasing fresh foods that do not contain genetic modifications, thereby supporting natural eating methods.

Freshness

- Consumers should select fresh, unprocessed foods before highly processed products in order to obtain optimal nutrients.

- The practice of eating seasonal produce helps consumers to select fresh items with better nutrient content.

Tips for Maintaining Balance

Meal Planning and Preparation

Plan Ahead

- Make a weekly planner with the incorporated balance of alkaline and acidic foods.

- A shopping list created according to the planned meals helps you acquire all essential ingredients.

Meal Prep

- Making large portions of meals initially and then dividing them into portions for the entire week limits both preparation time and ensures daily balanced meals.

- Moist foods must be kept in the refrigerator or freezer, while prepped foods require storage for maintaining freshness alongside convenience.

Hydration

Importance of Water

- Regular hydration through daily water drinking helps support pH equilibrium while maintaining body hydration levels.

- Drinking water that contains lemon and cucumber or berry slices can give you hydration and alkalinizing properties.

Herbal Teas

- You should trade sodas and sugary drinks with herbal tea as this beverage offers hydration as well as nutritional benefits.

Mindful Eating

Focus on Food

- Meals should be enjoyed without interruptions while you digest your food for better satisfaction.

- Plotting Your Body Signals against Hunger and Fullness Helps Both Control Quantity Consumed and Maintain Dietary Balance.

Portion Control

- The plate method should be used to split food into appropriate sections containing vegetables and proteins alongside grains.

- Small pots help control food serving sizes by allowing you to visualize portions more accurately to limit overeating.

Regular Monitoring and Adjustment

Check pH Levels

- You should test your urine pH levels with strips to know when to modify your eating habits.

- You should monitor your food consumption with pH level tracking through a food diary to detect eating patterns that need dietary changes.

Health Assessments

- Make sure to set appointments for medical tests that will track your general health situation together with nutritional indicators.

- Follow Medical Experts by Getting Periodic Blood Analyses to Identify Nutrient Levels and Fix Any Found Deficiencies.

Conclusion

Proper implementation of pH-balanced diets needs personalized nutritional review alongside balanced nutrition planning and attention to food quality. The maintenance of balanced pH and good health results from planning meals while practicing mindful eating and staying hydrated while conducting regular health checks. A comprehensive nutrition philosophy emphasizes maintaining health through mindful dietary choices.

Integrating Superfoods into Daily Meals

Strong health advantages stem from superfoods containing high levels of essential nutrients while providing numerous vitamins, minerals, antioxidants, and other required substances. The healthcare professional teaches patients that using superfoods regularly in their food consumption will result in better health outcomes. This guide presents daily usage methods for superfoods while showing productive examples for breakfast, lunch, dinner, snacks, and beverages.

Understanding Superfoods

The category of whole foods without refinement contains numerous nutrients in very high concentrations. Consuming superfoods delivers beneficial effects, such as strengthening immunity while providing increased energy and supporting cardiovascular health alongside better digestion and a better mental state. Berries and leafy greens, nuts and seeds, and fatty fish with fermented foods comprise the list of well-known superfoods.

12. Superfoods for Daily Meals

Breakfast

Smoothie Bowls

- Ingredients: Spinach, kale, blueberries, chia seeds, almond milk, banana

- The nutrient content in these foods includes antioxidants with fiber and vitamins that create beneficial effects for detoxification and provide energy to the body.

- Recipe: Blend spinach, kale, blueberries, banana, and almond milk until smooth. Transfer the mixture into a bowl, then decorate it with sliced bananas, followed by chia seeds and gathered nuts.

Oatmeal

- Ingredients: Oats, flaxseeds, walnuts, cinnamon, fresh berries, almond milk

- The nut mix contains essential nutrients for sustaining energy while supporting heart health through antioxidants, omega-3 fatty acids, and dietary fiber.

- Recipe: Cook oats in almond milk. Stir in flaxseeds and cinnamon. Place the dish under fresh berries and chopped walnuts.

Lunch

Quinoa Salad

- Ingredients: Quinoa, avocado, cherry tomatoes, cucumbers, chickpeas, spinach, olive oil, lemon juice

- This meal offers many health factors, including protein, healthy fat, fiber, and antioxidants, which promote digestive and heart wellness.

•	Follow the pack instructions to cook quinoa. Place cooked quinoa with diced avocado and tomatoes into a big mixing bowl. Add in cucumber, chickpeas, and spinach. Mix olive oil and lemon juice over the ingredients before blending everything together.

Superfood Wrap

•	You will need whole grain tortilla wrap, prepared hummus, a mix of fresh greens, pulled carrots, chopped red peppers, alfalfa sprouts, and sunflower seeds.

•	Benefits: Packed with vitamins, minerals, and antioxidants for immune support and energy.

•	Recipe: Spread hummus on a whole-grain wrap. Place fresh mixed greens on the wrap first, then top them with shredded carrots, sliced red bell peppers, sprouts, and sunflower seeds. Roll up and enjoy.

Dinner

Salmon and Veggie Stir-Fry

•	Ingredients: Salmon, broccoli, bell peppers, garlic, ginger, quinoa, sesame oil, tamari sauce

•	These foods provide omega-3 fatty acids, protein antioxidants, and fiber that help maintain heart health and lower inflammation.

•	Following package directions, cook quinoa until ready. Heat sesame oil in a frying pan, then add minced garlic and ginger. Combine broccoli and peppers in the pan, then stir-fry until all veggies become tender. Put salmon in the pan and let it cook until it reaches the proper state. Sprinkle tamari sauce over cooked quinoa to serve it as the base.

Lentil and Sweet Potato Curry

•	Ingredients: Lentils, sweet potatoes, spinach, coconut milk, curry powder, turmeric, garlic, ginger

•	Benefits: Rich in protein, fiber, vitamins, and anti-inflammatory compounds.

- Heat minced garlic and ginger in a large cooking pot. Stir the spices in curry powder and turmeric into the pot for one minute of cooking. Stir lentils with diced sweet potatoes and pour coconut milk into the pan. Continue to cook until both lentils and sweet potatoes become soft. Stir in spinach until wilted. Enjoy this dish with either brown rice or quinoa as your base.

Snacks

Greek Yogurt with Berries and Nuts

- Ingredients: Greek yogurt, blueberries, raspberries, almonds, honey

- Greek yogurt with blueberries, raspberries, almonds, and honey helps build digestive wellness and boosts energy with probiotics, protein, antioxidants, and healthy fat.

- Mix Greek yogurt with blueberries and raspberries into one bowl. Spread chopped almonds across the yogurt and pour honey over it.

Veggie Sticks with Hummus

- Hungry eaters should combine carrot sticks, cucumber slices, and bell pepper strips with a hummus dip for their plate.

- The food combination offers important plant compounds that strengthen your immune system and provide you with energy.

- To enjoy your meal, provide a selection of raw veggies with a separate portion of hummus for dipping.

Beverages

Green Smoothie

- Ingredients: Spinach, kale, cucumber, green apple, lemon, ginger, coconut water

- Benefits: Rich in chlorophyll, vitamins, and antioxidants for detoxification and energy.

- Recipe: Blend spinach, kale, cucumber, green apple, lemon juice, ginger, and coconut water until smooth. Pour into a glass and enjoy.

Turmeric Latte

- Ingredients: Turmeric, ginger, cinnamon, almond milk, honey

- It helps protect the immune system and decreases inflammation because of its antioxidant and anti-inflammatory qualities.

- Recipe: In a saucepan, heat almond milk with turmeric, ginger, and cinnamon. Stir all ingredients and warm the mixture until everything blends well. Sweeten with honey to taste.

Integrating Superfoods Seamlessly

Plan Ahead

- Prepare your meals ahead of time to regularly include superfoods in your meals.

- Make a buying list that contains many superfood products to keep your supply of them steady.

Experiment with Recipes

- Add superfoods to new recipe experiments to create better meals for eating.

- Include superfoods in your regular favorite meals. Make chia seeds a topping for your cereal dish, and stir spinach into your pasta sauce.

Balanced Approach

- Include multiple types of superfoods in your meals to get all needed nutrients from the diet.

- Having superfoods once a day helps, but you should blend them with regular healthy foods to create an even diet.

Conclusion

Using superfoods as part of your regular diet will help boost your health naturally. Your immune health and mental wellness will improve as well, and your digestive system and heart will get stronger when you eat nutrition-packed foods at every meal. Dietary balance in nutrition emphasizes the inclusion of superfoods to support overall health and well-being.

Superfoods for Breakfast, Lunch, Dinner, Snacks, Beverages

Adding superfoods consistently to your meals will improve your total health results. Superfoods play a crucial role in nutrition by providing abundant vitamins, minerals, antioxidants, and essential plant nutrients that support overall health and well-being. This guide offers real examples of what to eat, including superfoods at breakfast, lunch, dinner, snack, and drink times.

Superfoods for Breakfast

Smoothie Bowls

A meal of spinach, kale with blueberries, and chia seeds combined with banana and almond milk brings essential antioxidants, vitamins, and fiber for better energy performance. Recipe: Blend spinach, kale, blueberries, banana, and almond milk until smooth. Settle the mixture inside a serving bowl, and then decorate it with chia seeds, banana slices, and crushed nuts.

Oatmeal with Superfoods

Ingredients: Oats, flaxseeds, walnuts, cinnamon, fresh berries, almond milk Benefits: Provides fiber, omega-3 fatty acids, and antioxidants for heart health and sustained energy. Recipe: Cook oats in almond milk. Stir in flaxseeds and cinnamon. Set almonds and fresh berries on top of the mixture.

Avocado Toast

Ingredients: Whole grain bread, avocado, chia seeds, cherry tomatoes, olive oil, lemon juice.

Benefits: High in healthy fats, fiber, and antioxidants. Apply mashed avocado onto whole grain bread for the meal preparation. Use olive oil to dress the mixture before sprinkling it with chia seeds and topping it with cherry tomato slices and lemon juice.

Superfoods for Lunch

Quinoa Salad

The mix of quinoa, avocado, tomato, cucumber chickpea, spinach, olive oil, and lemon juice offers protein, fiber, healthy fat, and antioxidants for healthy digestion and heart functions. Follow these directions to make quinoa: Prepare the ingredients based on the instructions on the product packaging. Place all items, such as cooked quinoa and diced vegetables, into a big mixing container. Lightly pour olive oil and lemon juice over the mix before mixing everything together.

Superfood Wrap

The combination of whole grain wrap with hummus topping plus a mix of greens and colorful veggies, along with sprouts and sunflower seeds, offers you many vitamins and antioxidants that boost your immune system and give you energy. Recipe: Spread hummus on a whole-grain wrap. Build your wrap with spinach leaves, then add shredded carrots, red bell pepper slices, sunflower seeds, and sprouts. Roll up and enjoy.

Lentil Soup

Ingredients: Lentils, carrots, celery, onions, garlic, turmeric, spinach, vegetable broth. Benefits: Rich in protein, fiber, vitamins, and anti-inflammatory compounds. Recipe: Sauté onions, garlic, and celery in olive oil until soft. Stir turmeric into the mixture for one minute. Stew lentils and vegetable broth until the lentils become soft. Stir in spinach until wilted.

Superfoods for Dinner

Salmon and Veggie Stir-Fry

Ingredients: Salmon, broccoli, bell peppers, garlic, ginger, quinoa, sesame oil, tamari sauce Benefits: Provides omega-3 fatty acids, protein, antioxidants, and fiber for heart health and inflammation reduction. Prepare quinoa by using the directions provided by the manufacturer. Put sesame oil in a skillet and add minced garlic and ginger to it. Combine broccoli and bell peppers with the pan and cook until soft. Put salmon portions into the pan, and then cook until they reach the desired state. Season the dish with tamari sauce, and then enjoy it over quinoa.

Lentil and Sweet Potato Curry

Ingredients: Lentils, sweet potatoes, spinach, coconut milk, curry powder, turmeric, garlic, ginger. Benefits: Rich in protein, fiber, vitamins, and anti-inflammatory compounds. Put minced garlic and ginger into a big pot before starting to cook. Cook curry powder and turmeric for one minute. Combine lentils with diced sweet potatoes and coconut milk into the pot. Cook the mixture until both lentils and sweet potatoes become soft. Stir in spinach until wilted. Serve the dish with brown rice or quinoa as the base.

Chickpea and Spinach Stew

Ingredients: Chickpeas, spinach, tomatoes, onions, garlic, cumin, coriander, olive oil. Benefits: High in protein, fiber, vitamins, and minerals. Recipe: Sauté onions and garlic in olive oil until soft. Cook the combination of cumin and coriander for one minute. Place chickpeas and tomatoes into the pan before simmering it for twenty minutes. Stir in spinach until wilted.

Superfoods for Snacks

Greek Yogurt with Berries and Nuts

Ingredients: Greek yogurt, blueberries, raspberries, almonds, honey Benefits: Provides probiotics, protein, antioxidants, and healthy fats for digestive health and sustained energy. Blend Greek yogurt with blueberries alongside raspberries into a bowl for this snack. Finish the creation with chopped almonds alongside a drop of honey.

Veggie Sticks with Hummus

The following snack contains carrot sticks, cucumber slices together, and bell pepper strips served with hummus while providing essential fiber, vitamins, minerals, and beneficial, healthy fats to support immune function and boost energy levels. Two options for a snack include presenting vegetable sticks with hummus as a dip.

Almonds and Dark Chocolate

Ingredients: Almonds, dark chocolate (70% cocoa or higher) Benefits: Provides healthy fats, antioxidants, and a satisfying, nutrient-dense snack. Users should mix almonds together with dark chocolate pieces to make an equal snack serving.

Superfoods for Beverages

Green Smoothie

Ingredients: Spinach, kale, cucumber, green apple, lemon, ginger, coconut water Benefits: Rich in chlorophyll, vitamins, and antioxidants for detoxification and energy. Recipe: Blend spinach, kale, cucumber, green apple, lemon juice, ginger, and coconut water until smooth. Pour into a glass and enjoy.

Turmeric Latte

You need turmeric together with ginger, cinnamon, almond milk, and honey to make this drink, which gives your immune health support and inflammation reduction benefits. Recipe: In a saucepan, heat almond milk with turmeric, ginger, and cinnamon. Stir the mixture while heat brings the solution to a combined consistency. Sweeten with honey to taste.

Chia Seed Lemon Water

The mixture of Chia seeds and lemon juice combined with water contains optional honey and provides hydration plus dietary fiber, omega-3 fatty acids, and antioxidant properties. To create this recipe, soak chia seeds in a glass of water for a period of 10-15 minutes. Pour lemon juice along with honey through personal preference. Stir well and drink.

Conclusion

Daily consumption of superfoods leads to improved health since their nutrients support complete wellness. Different healthy foods consumed during breakfast, lunch, dinner, snacks, and beverages enhance both your immune system health and your energy levels and heart wellness, along with gut health benefits and enhanced mental wellness. A nutritional approach that emphasizes superfoods promotes health benefits through a balanced diet incorporating a variety of nutrient-dense food categories.

Integrating Superfoods Seamlessly

Making superfoods a part of your daily dietary intake proves simple as well as pleasant. Your diet gets better when you add nutritious foods that effectively support your complete health improvement. The guide offers step-by-step guidelines along with strategies to help you naturally add superfoods to your food without any difficulty for maximum health advantages.

Practical Tips for Integrating Superfoods

Plan Ahead

An important strategy to maintain superfoods in your diet is to organize meals during preparation time. The shopping list must contain different superfoods to help maintain a fully stocked pantry.

Experiment with Recipes

People should test different meal recipes, which include superfoods, to discover both enjoyable and nutritious options. You should put superfoods into your favorite recipes to modify them. Chia seeds make an excellent topping for cereal, while spinach can be blended into pasta sauce.

Balanced Approach

Children should build their diet around several different superfoods because this helps meet their requirements for essential nutrients. The advantages of superfoods should be managed through a balanced diet approach with other nutritious foods needed to achieve overall dietary equilibrium.

Breakfast

Smoothie Bowls

Ingredients: Spinach, kale, blueberries, chia seeds, almond milk, banana. How to Integrate: Blend spinach, kale, blueberries, banana, and almond milk until smooth. A bowl should receive the blended mixture while chia seeds, sliced bananas, and a small portion of nuts provide decoration on top. This food provides health benefits through its antioxidant content along with fiber and vital nutrient combination, which aids in energy production and detoxification processes.

Oatmeal with Superfoods

The breakfast ingredient list contains oats, flaxseeds, walnuts, cinnamon, and fresh berries with almond milk. The preparation process consists of cooking oats by using almond milk. Stir in flaxseeds and cinnamon. Place the serving dish on top with fresh berries and chopped walnuts. Eating this meal gives you three important health benefits because it contains fiber, omega-3 fatty acids, and antioxidants that enhance heart health and provide sustained energy levels.

Avocado Toast

The nutritional components of this recipe start with whole grain bread and continue with avocado, followed by chia seeds together with cherry tomatoes using olive oil and lemon juice. Set the dish with chia seeds on top and cherry tomato slices, and drizzle olive oil with lemon juice squeezed onto the mix. Benefits: High in healthy fats, fiber, and antioxidants.

Lunch

Quinoa Salad

The needed ingredients include Quinoa along with avocado and cherry tomatoes with cut cucumbers and chickpeas with spinach while utilizing olive oil and lemon juice. A mixture of cooked quinoa along with diced avocado combines with cherry tomatoes and cucumbers while incorporating chickpeas and spinach in a large bowl. The mixture requires olive oil and lemon juice, which you should combine by tossing the ingredients together. This dish provides an excellent combination of protein with healthy fats, fiber, and antioxidants that help your digestive system work well and support heart health.

Superfood Wrap

Prepare the wrap by applying hummus to a whole-grain base. Place whole grain wraps by spreading hummus, then continue with mixed greens, shredded carrots, sliced red bell peppers, sprouts, and sunflower seeds. Roll up and enjoy. Benefits: Packed with vitamins, minerals, and antioxidants for immune support and energy.

Lentil Soup

Ingredients: Lentils, carrots, celery, onions, garlic, turmeric, spinach, vegetable broth. How to Integrate: Sauté onions, garlic, and celery in olive oil until soft. Continue to cook the mixture with turmeric for one minute. Put lentils into the pot with vegetable broth before allowing the lentils to become soft. Stir in spinach until wilted. Benefits: Rich in protein, fiber, vitamins, and anti-inflammatory compounds.

Dinner

Salmon and Veggie Stir-Fry

The recipe requires Salmon, broccoli, bell peppers, garlic, ginger, and quinoa together with sesame oil and tamari sauce. Follow these steps: Prepare the quinoa as directed in the package. A pan filled with sesame oil requires heating, followed by minced garlic and minced ginger. Stir the vegetables, broccoli, and bell peppers in the pan until they become soft. The salmon needs to be added to the pan for completion. First, combine quinoa with tamari sauce and present it as the final course. Consuming this dish delivers three important benefits: omega-3 fatty acids, protein, antioxidants, and fiber, which strengthen heart function while reducing inflammation.

Lentil and Sweet Potato Curry

To make this recipe, start by placing minced garlic and ginger in a large pot, where you will sauté. Clarify the mixture with curry powder and turmeric before cooking for one minute. Transfer the ingredients of lentils and diced sweet potatoes along with coconut milk into the pot. Prolong cooking until the lentils, together with sweet potatoes, turn tender. Stir in spinach until wilted. Heat the dish with brown rice or quinoa as the base. Benefits: Rich in protein, fiber, vitamins, and anti-inflammatory compounds.

Chickpea and Spinach Stew

The necessary components for this dish are chickpeas alongside spinach, tomatoes, and onions with garlic accompanied by cumin, coriander powder, and olive oil. Preparation steps include sautéing onions and garlic in olive oil until they become tender. The mixture requires 1 minute of sautéing after adding cumin and coriander. The stew requires chickpeas and tomatoes, which should be cooked together for 20 minutes until ready. Stir in spinach until wilted. Benefits: High in protein, fiber, vitamins, and minerals.

Snacks

Greek Yogurt with Berries and Nuts

Greek yogurt serves as the base for this dish, along with blueberries, raspberries, almonds, and honey, which are secondary ingredients. All the components are combined in one bowl. Serve this dish by adding chopped almonds followed by a sweetening touch of honey. This meal contains probiotics together with protein antioxidants and healthy fats that help digestion and provide sustained energy benefits.

Veggie Sticks with Hummus

The recipe combines carrot sticks, cucumber slices, and bell pepper strips alongside hummus, which serves as a dipping sauce. This snack combination includes fiber as well as vitamins, minerals, and healthy fats, which help strengthen your immune system and provide sustained energy.

Almonds and Dark Chocolate

The necessary components for this treat are almonds and dark chocolate, which should contain 70% cocoa or more. Prepare it by uniting a small serving of almonds with two pieces of dark chocolate. Consuming these items will deliver necessary antioxidants together with healthy fats and offer satisfying dietary content.

Beverages

Green Smoothie

Ingredients: Spinach, kale, cucumber, green apple, lemon, ginger, coconut water. How to Integrate: Blend spinach, kale, cucumber, green apple, lemon juice, ginger, and coconut water until smooth. Pour into a glass and enjoy. Benefits: Rich in chlorophyll, vitamins, and antioxidants for detoxification and energy.

Turmeric Latte

Ingredients: Turmeric, ginger, cinnamon, almond milk, honey. How to Integrate: In a saucepan, heat almond milk with turmeric, ginger, and cinnamon. Stir the mixture until all components blend while heating it to the appropriate temperature. Sweeten with honey to taste. The combination of anti-inflammatory agents and antioxidants inside this mixture supports immune health and reduces inflammation.

Chia Seed Lemon Water

The preparation includes Chia seeds and a combination of lemon juice and water with an optional addition of honey. The integration process consists of mixing the ingredients together before leaving them to soak for 10-15 minutes. Add lemon juice together with honey at your preferred strength of flavor. Stir well and drink. The mixture contains hydrating properties with dietary fiber content and omega-3 acids together with antioxidant substances.

Conclusion

Using superfoods for daily meals becomes simple through both strategic planning and inventive thinking. Nutrient-dense ingredients from these foods can be added to every mealtime, including breakfast, lunch, dinner, and snacks and beverages, improving personal wellness. Nutrition plans that address both dietary needs and overall health emphasize balanced meals incorporating superfoods to enhance well-being.

13. Overcoming Digestive Disorders

Digestive disorders have a substantial influence on life quality that leads to multiple health problems, including gastrointestinal pain and insufficient nutrient intake. Managing digestive disorders involves dietary modifications, lifestyle adjustments, and the use of natural remedies to promote optimal gut health and overall well-being. The guide features methods and approaches to handle standard digestive medical problems while supporting intestinal wellness.

Signs and Symptoms of Common Digestive Issues

Common Digestive Disorders

1. **Irritable Bowel Syndrome (IBS)**

- The illness presents with these signs: Abdominal pain accompanies bloating together with gas, followed by both diarrhea and constipation.

- High-stress episodes and particular food products and natural hormonal modifications serve as activators leading to symptoms.

2. **Gastroesophageal Reflux Disease (GERD)**

- The signs and symptoms include heartburn with acid reflux together with chest discomfort, and swallowing problems.

- Triggers: Spicy foods, fatty foods, caffeine, alcohol

3. **Inflammatory Bowel Disease (IBD)**

- Symptoms: Chronic diarrhea, abdominal pain, weight loss, fatigue

- Types: Crohn's disease, ulcerative colitis

4. Constipation

- The symptoms of this condition include reduced bowel movements and hard stools, which result in the uncomfortable passing of stool.

- Triggers: Low fiber diet, dehydration, lack of physical activity

5. Diverticulitis

- Symptoms: Abdominal pain, fever, nausea, changes in bowel habits

- Low fiber diet, together with age and obesity, act as triggers for this condition.

Recognizing Symptoms

- The abdomen expands into a swollen feeling with fullness, which is termed as bloating.

- Gas: Excessive belching or flatulence

- Diarrhea: Frequent, loose, or watery stools

- Constipation: Infrequent or difficult bowel movements

- Stomach pain that cramps or causes discomfort in the area below the waist constitutes one symptom of digestive disorder.

Herbal and Dietary Interventions for Digestive Disorders

Herbal Remedies

1. Ginger

- The use of ginger provides three main benefits, including the reduction of nausea, better digestion, and active anti-inflammatory properties.

- Fresh ginger tea, ginger capsules, and fresh ginger in meals remain the recommended ways to use this remedy.

2. **Peppermint**

- The intake of peppermint provides multiple advantages, including symptom relief for IBS patients while reducing pain for abdominal discomfort and bowel distension.

- Usage: Peppermint tea, enteric-coated peppermint oil capsules

3. **Chamomile**

- Benefits: Soothes the digestive tract, reduces inflammation and spasms

- Usage: Chamomile tea, chamomile extract

4. **Turmeric**

- This spice reveals two main characteristics: inflammation reduction ability and protection for digestive health.

- The recommended usage of turmeric includes making tea with the spice, taking capsules, and adding the spice to regular meals.

5. **Slippery Elm**

- The medicinal value of slippery elm includes protective and calming properties for the digestive tract in addition to its anti-inflammatory effects.

- Slippery elm powder needs the addition of water to create a mixture, or consumers can take slippery elm lozenges.

Dietary Interventions

1. **High-Fiber Diet**

- Consuming slippery elm has two beneficial effects, which include normalizing bowel movements while protecting against constipation.

- Sources: Whole grains, fruits, vegetables, legumes, nuts, seeds

2. **Probiotics**

•   Consuming slippery elm provides two main benefits: normalizing gut bacteria populations while supporting digestive health.

•   Sources: Yogurt, kefir, sauerkraut, kimchi, miso, probiotic supplements

3. **Prebiotics**

•   The consumption of beneficial probiotics through prebiotics allows people to feed beneficial gut bacteria and significantly improves their gut health.

•   Sources: Garlic, onions, leeks, asparagus, bananas, chicory root

4. **Hydration**

•   Benefits: Essential for digestion and preventing constipation

•   Hydration sources include drinking plenty of water together with eating water-filled foods such as cucumbers and watermelon.

5. **Anti-Inflammatory Foods**

•   Benefits: Reduce inflammation in the digestive tract

•   Sources: Berries, leafy greens, nuts, fatty fish, olive oil

Foods to Avoid

1. **Processed Foods**

•   Issues: Contain additives, preservatives, and low in nutrients

•   Fast food, together with packaged snacks and sugary cereals, represent examples of these problematic food items.

2. **Fried and Fatty Foods**

•   The digestive process makes these foods hard to break down, and GERD and IBS symptoms might crop up as a result.

- French fries alongside fried chicken paired with heavy cream sauces constitute examples of foods that should be avoided.

3. Dairy Products

- Having dairy products triggers diarrhea and bloating symptoms in people with lactose intolerance.
- Alternatives: Plant-based milk, lactose-free dairy products

4. Caffeine and Alcohol

- Physical therapy from these ingredients creates an irritated digestive system which intensifies symptoms.
- Alternatives: Herbal teas, water, non-caffeinated beverages

5. Spicy Foods

- This dietary item causes heartburn and acid reflux as its side effects.
- Dry spices or gentle plant extracts represent suitable replacement ingredients for the avoidance of spicy food.

Lifestyle Changes for Gut Health Improvement

Regular Physical Activity

- Regular bowel movements, together with a reduction of stress and support of overall health, are benefits derived from this action.
- People with IBS should perform walking, jogging, yoga, swimming, and cycling along with physical activities.

Stress Management

- Regular consumption of herbal tea combined with water along with non-caffeinated fluids helps decrease digestive system stress.
- Techniques: Meditation, deep breathing exercises, mindfulness, yoga, tai chi

Adequate Sleep

- The practice of physical exercise leads to multiple advantages that support body health and stress reduction and promote better digestion functions.

- The implementation of a routine sleep schedule and a relaxed bedtime ritual, along with keeping screens away from bedtime, helps to reduce stress-related bowel problems.

Mindful Eating

- Benefits: Improves digestion, reduces overeating, promotes better food choices

- Techniques: Eat slowly, chew thoroughly, avoid distractions during meals

Routine and Regularity

- Benefits: Establishes regular bowel habits, supports digestive health

- Tips: Eat meals at consistent times, establish a regular bathroom routine

Conclusion

A successful treatment approach for digestive disorders includes the integration of herbal medicines, eating carefully considered diets, and making beneficial life changes. Digestive disorders can be managed through dietary choices of high-fiber foods and probiotics with anti-inflammatory properties, together with measures to avoid trigger foods and maintain healthy life habits. A holistic approach to digestive health emphasizes balanced, mindful, and diverse eating habits, promoting overall well-being and improved gut function.

14. Managing Diabetes Naturally

Diabetes management through natural methods requires a complete approach in which people should follow dietary modifications along with exercise routines, herbal solutions, and lifestyle modifications. Natural methods serve as the foundation for supporting overall health and maintaining balanced blood sugar levels. This approach emphasizes nutrition, lifestyle adjustments, and holistic wellness strategies. This document offers applicable approaches for handling diabetes through natural methods.

Understanding the Role of Diet in Diabetes

The dietary choices people make contribute essential management of diabetes. A person can sustain stable blood sugar levels and promote better health by eating whole foods instead of processed foods in a balanced diet.

Key Dietary Principles

1. Low Glycemic Index Foods

- Through their consumption, people can maintain stable blood sugar levels as they slow down sugar absorption spikes.

- Examples: Whole grains, legumes, vegetables, fruits (berries, apples, pears), nuts, seeds.

2. High-Fiber Foods

- These foods provide two advantages, which are to delay sugar absorption while keeping your digestive system healthy.

- Examples: Oats, barley, quinoa, brown rice, vegetables, legumes, and fruits (apples, oranges, berries).

3. **Healthy Fats**

- Insulin sensitivity improves when people eat foods containing these foods because they deliver sustained energy.

- Examples: Avocados, nuts, seeds, olive oil, fatty fish (salmon, mackerel).

4. **Lean Proteins**

- The advantages of lean proteins and muscles include their ability to maintain body tissues while preventing blood sugar spikes.

- Examples of these proteins include chicken, turkey, fish, legumes, tofu, and eggs.

5. **Minimize Processed Foods and Sugars**

- The consumption of this diet lowers blood sugar spikes and minimizes overall body inflammation.

- The following foods should be avoided: sugary snacks as well as sodas with refined grains and processed foods.

Key Herbs for Blood Sugar Regulation

Natural herbal substances function to stabilize blood sugar levels while promoting stable health. Several medical herbs demonstrate effectiveness in diabetes management through various research studies.

1. **Cinnamon**

- The consumption of cinnamon leads to improved insulin sensitivity together with reduced blood sugar concentration.

- Usage: Add ground cinnamon to smoothies, oatmeal, and tea.

2. **Fenugreek**

- Implementation of fenugreek brings delayed carbohydrate absorption with enhanced insulin sensitivity as advantages to the body.

- The practice of soaking fenugreek seeds in water overnight will result in consumable water in the morning, whereas adding fenugreek powder to meals works similarly.

3. **Berberine**

- The consumption of cinnamon provides two health advantages: it lowers blood sugar and boosts insulin sensitivity.

- Follow the recommended dosing of berberine supplements that your healthcare provider will give you.

4. **Bitter Melon**

- This compound in the plant shows the ability to decrease blood sugar levels.

- You can drink bitter melon juice or consume supplement forms of the melon.

5. **Aloe Vera**

- Benefits: Improves blood sugar control and reduces inflammation.

- Usage: Consume aloe vera juice or gel.

6. **Gymnema Sylvestre**

- The consumption of Gymnema pseudopanax leads to lower sugar intake in the intestines while making insulin perform better.

- After judgment, one can take Gymnema supplements alongside drinking Gymnema tea.

General Guidelines for Taking Herbs for Blood Sugar Regulation

- A healthcare professional needs to evaluate all herbal treatments before starting since people who take medication for diabetes should receive special attention.

- Begin with small amounts of herbal medication to observe body reactions before continuing your dosage at desired levels.

- Blood sugar level monitoring must stay consistent to verify that the herbal substances produce their expected effects.

- The best outcomes emerge from taking the herbal remedies every day with consistent adherence to a schedule.

Incorporating Exercise for Diabetes Management

The proper management of diabetes requires regular physical exercise since this physical activity enhances insulin sensitivity while improving overall health conditions.

Types of Exercise

1. **Aerobic Exercise**

- Benefits: Increases cardiovascular health and improves insulin sensitivity.

- Examples: Walking, jogging, cycling, swimming.

2. **Resistance Training**

- Benefits: Builds musclemass and improves insulin sensitivity.

- Weight lifting combined with resistance bands along with push-ups and squats makes up good exercise examples for this category.

3. **Flexibility and Balance Exercises**

- Exercising improves mobility and simultaneously cuts down chances for accidents.

- Three examples of these exercises include Yoga, tai chi, and stretching exercises.

Exercise Guidelines

• To obtain health benefits engage in moderate aerobic exercises totaling at least 150 minutes throughout a minimum of seven days per week.

• Intensity: Include both moderate and vigorous-intensity exercises.

• Consistency plays an essential role when you establish exercise as a permanent element of your daily life.

• Each workout requires blood sugar monitoring before exercise and after exercise particularly when you use insulin or take blood sugar-lowering medications.

Lifestyle Changes for Diabetes Management

Stress Management

• Stress poses two related dangers for diabetic patients because it increases blood sugar and interferes with diabetes management.

• The practice of relaxation techniques includes meditation combined with deep breathing exercises together with yoga and mindfulness as effective methods.

Adequate Sleep

• The control of blood sugar, together with total health stability, becomes adversely impacted when sleep deteriorates.

• Your routine for better sleep involves scheduling regular rest times, building relaxing nighttime processes, and ensuring relaxed sleeping conditions.

Hydration

• The benefits of hydration include proper blood sugar management, together with general health maintenance.

- The recommended advice includes drinking water all day while limiting sugary beverages and adding cucumber and watermelon to your hydration diet.

Regular Monitoring

- Checking your blood sugar levels frequently allows you to learn which foods and activities combined with stress affect your diabetes condition.

- The tools you need include the blood glucose meter together with the continuous glucose monitor (CGM) or additional devices that your healthcare professional will recommend.

Conclusion

People who want to manage diabetes naturally must make food adjustments while using herbal remedies as well as exercise regularly and restructure their daily routines. Your blood sugar control and your general health improvement can be achieved through balanced eating combined with herbal medicines, physical exercise, and stress management practices. A comprehensive system utilizing natural healthcare techniques supports sustainable wellness for individuals managing diabetes. This approach integrates nutrition, lifestyle modifications, and holistic health strategies to promote long-term well-being.

15. Heart Health and Hypertension

Proper heart health management, along with successful hypertension control requirements, sustains both life expectancy and general health effectiveness. Achieving optimal heart health and managing blood pressure effectively requires a whole-person approach that integrates nutritional adjustments, lifestyle improvements, and complementary health strategies. This comprehensive method promotes long-term cardiovascular well-being. The document delivers functional techniques to support heart wellness together with natural hypertension control methods.

Essential Heart Health Nutrients and Herbs

Nutrients for Heart Health

1. **Omega-3 Fatty Acids**

• Oily fish, together with seeds and nuts as sources, provide four cardinal benefits, which include inflammation reduction and blood pressure regulation alongside triglyceride management and cardiovascular wellness.

• Sources: Fatty fish (salmon, mackerel, sardines), flaxseeds, chia seeds, walnuts.

2. **Fiber**

• Fiber consumption creates dual health benefits because it controls blood sugar levels and reduces cholesterol yet maintains excellent satiety to help people maintain their weight.

• The dietary intake should include whole grains together with fruits, vegetables, and legumes, along with nuts and seeds.

3. **Potassium**

•   Consuming potassium can regulate blood pressure because it balances sodium while supporting heart operation.

•   Sources: Bananas, oranges, potatoes, spinach, avocados.

4. **Magnesium**

•   the heart obtains a normal rhythm through this nutrient, which controls blood pressure at the same time, it maintains muscle and nerve function.

•   The recommended food sources include seeds and nuts, in addition to whole grains, along with leafy green vegetables.

5. **Antioxidants**

•   Heart protection from oxidative stress and heart-damaging inflammation occurs when people incorporate this food into their diet.

•   Sources: Berries, dark chocolate, nuts, green tea, leafy greens.

Herbs for Heart Health

1. **Hawthorn**

•   Hawthorn bends blood flow better while reducing blood pressure pressure and making heart muscle stronger.

•   Usage: Hawthorn tea, capsules, or tinctures.

2. **Garlic**

•   The health benefits of this substance include blood pressure reduction as well as cholesterol level reduction alongside anti-inflammatory effects.

•   Usage: Fresh garlic, garlic supplements, or garlic oil.

3. **Turmeric**

- Benefits: Anti-inflammatory properties support cardiovascular health.

- Turmeric tea and turmeric capsules and the use of turmeric in food items serve as the recommended usage of this supplement.

4. **Cayenne Pepper**

- This herb offers multiple advantages which consist of promoting blood flow and decreasing high blood pressure while providing antioxidant benefits to the body.

- The usage of cayenne pepper capsules or food administration with this pepper is allowed in prevention strategies.

5. **Ginger**

- Using these herbs provides three benefits: inflammation reduction, improved circulation, and blood pressure regulation.

- The consumption of fresh ginger tea along with ginger capsules and meals that include fresh ginger constitutes usage methods for the benefits.

Diet and Lifestyle for Blood Pressure Management

Dietary Recommendations

1. **DASH Diet (Dietary Approaches to Stop Hypertension)**

- A core element of DASH principles requires members to eat mainly whole grains along with vegetables combined with lean proteins, fruits, and low-fat dairy foods while simultaneously eating reduced sodium amounts.

- The DASH Diet provides medical evidence that it controls blood pressure in addition to defending cardiovascular well-being.

2.   **Reduce Sodium Intake**

•   New research indicates that daily sodium consumption should not exceed 2,300 mg, but people should actively work toward reaching 1,500 mg daily targets.

•   Breakfast Foods Prevented from Use Include processed foods together with canned soups as well as salty snacks. Herbs and spice mixtures prove a better choice for adding flavor rather than using salt.

3.   **Increase Potassium-Rich Foods**

•   Consuming potassium helps regulate sodium effects by sustaining heart health.

•   Sources: Bananas, oranges, potatoes, spinach, avocados.

4.   **Limit Alcohol Consumption**

•   Men should stay within two daily alcohol limits, with women following one daily limit.

•   Benefits: Reduces the risk of hypertension and other cardiovascular issues.

5.   **Healthy Fats**

•   The recommended dietary changes include consuming omega-3 fatty acids and monounsaturated fats as healthy fatty acids.

•   Sources: Fatty fish, avocados, olive oil, nuts, seeds.

6.   **Whole Grains**

•   Consuming fiber in food helps individuals regulate their blood pressure and cholesterol levels.

•   Sources: Brown rice, quinoa, whole wheat, oats.

Lifestyle Recommendations

1. Regular Physical Activity

It benefits heart health while helping people maintain their weight and control their blood pressure.

The recommendation for exercise duration should match 150 minutes per week of moderate-intensity aerobic exercises, which include brisk walking, jogging, or cycling.

2. Weight Management

- The heart and blood pressure experience fewer burdens when a person maintains their weight within healthy limits.

- The combination of proper nutrition and physical exercise serves as the recommendation to reach and sustain the ideal body weight.

3. Stress Management

- Regular practice of stress management techniques enables people to protect their cardiovascular system from harm while lowering their blood pressure readings.

- One should practice relaxation methods that include meditation along with deep breathing exercises in combination with yoga and mindfulness practice.

4. Quit Smoking

- The elimination of heart disease risk alongside better general health serves as one of the main advantages of this approach.

- The recommendation for smoking cessation support includes contacting healthcare experts or joining professional smoking cessation programs or support sessions.

5. Adequate Sleep

- Regular sleep maintains overall health and decreases stress together withblood pressure control.

- The recommended amount of quality sleep per night falls between 7 and 9 hours. People should establish routine sleep patterns alongside a calming preparation before bedtime.

Natural Solutions for Respiratory Conditions

Herbal Remedies for Asthma and Allergies

1. **Butterbur**

- Benefits: Reduces inflammation and smooth muscle spasms in the airways.

- Usage: Butterbur supplements or extracts.

2. **Quercetin**

- The substance works as a natural antihistamine to reduce allergic reactions.

- Quercetin supplements, together with apples, onions, and berries, provide two benefits: the supplements serve as natural antihistamines that reduce allergic reactions.

3. **Stinging Nettle**

- Benefits: Reduces symptoms of hay fever and allergies.

- The three methods of consuming nettle tea and capsules together with extracts are suitable for this treatment.

4. **Ginger**

- The use of ginger results in two main advantages fighting inflammation while relaxing the passageways.

- The recommended usages for ginger benefits include fresh ginger tea along with ginger capsules as well as eating meals that contain fresh ginger.

5. Licorice Root

•   Technical advantages of licorice roots include both respiratory tract soothing and anti-inflammatory effects.

•   The appropriate usage of licorice root occurs in its forms as tea and capsules or extracts.

Improving Respiratory Health Through Lifestyle

1. Avoiding Triggers

yönethe avoidance of both allergic substances and respiratory triggers such as dust particles, smoke pollen grains, and pet fur microorganisms.

2. Regular Exercise

•   Benefits: Improves lung function and overall respiratory health.

Rephrase this section: Moderate-intensity exercises involving walking, swimming, and cycling prove beneficial for therapeutic purposes.

3. Breathing Exercises

•   Designed breathing exercises enable people to strengthen their breathing muscles and build lung capacity.

•   There are three breathing exercises that provide benefits to lung health: deep breathing exercises, diaphragmatic breathing, and pursed-lip breathing.

4. Humidifiers

•   Moisture in the air helps minimize respiratory irritation across the space.

•   Usage: Use a humidifier in your home, especially during dry weather or winter months.

5. Healthy Diet

•   The consumption of this diet supports the health of your respiratory system while minimizing inflammation levels.

- To support respiratory health, patients should consume nutritious food that combines fruits with vegetables together with whole grains, lean proteins, and healthy fats.

Techniques to Enhance Air Quality at Home

1. Air Purifiers

- The use of air purifiers delivers many advantages by drawing allergens and dust along with pollutants out from indoor air.

- High-efficiency particulate air (HEPA) filters should be used to enhance indoor air quality.

2. Regular Cleaning

- Homeowners who adopt this technique minimize the buildup of airborne allergens along with mold and dust in their environment.

- The recommendation is to vacuum the floor continually and clean surfaces repeatedly along with frequent washing of bedding.

3. Ventilation

- Room air pollutants decrease while air movements increase when you implement this approach.

- Your home should have open windows and exhaust fans as well as sufficient ventilation.

4. Natural Cleaning Products

- Benefits: Reduces exposure to harsh chemicals and irritants.

- Recommendations: Use natural or non-toxic cleaning products.

Conclusion

To maintain heart health and control blood pressure you need to make a full range of changes to your diet, physical activity and lifestyle as well as use herbal remedies. Your cardiovascular health and blood pressure control better function when you eat nutritious foods, use herbal remedies, stay physically active, and reduce stress. The natural practices help people keep good health for a long period.

16. Natural Solutions for Respiratory Conditions

Patients with asthma allergies and other respiratory conditions can lead better lives through natural medications and improved lifestyles. This resource gives you tools to improve your respiratory health plus methods to control well-known respiratory problems.

Herbal Remedies for Asthma and Allergies

1. **Butterbur**

• The plant helps decrease airway swelling and stops muscle spasms within the bronchi.

• Usage: Butterbur supplements or extracts.

• You should only use butterbur products with zero pyrrolizidine alkaloids to avoid potential risks.

2. **Quercetin**

• Quercetin naturally fights allergic reactions as an antihistamine.

• Body tries to fight allergy symptoms better when you consume food items which contain quercetin including apples and onions plus take quercetin supplements.

3. **Stinging Nettle**

• The plant helps people who suffer from hay fever and allergic reactions.

• Consumers can take Nettle products either as tea or capsules.

4. **Ginger**

• The root works to decrease swelling and calms the breathing passages.

- People use fresh ginger tea drinks plus take capsules and add raw ginger to food.

5. **Licorice Root**

- The respiratory system and inflammation get softer when you use this product.

- People can use licorice root products such as tea and capsules for this therapy.

- You should take licorice root with care when you have hypertension.

6. **Mullein**

- The respiratory system feels better when users try this remedy because it thins mucus secretions.

- Usage: Mullein tea or tincture.

7. **Thyme**

- Thyme has natural antibiotics that fight respiratory infections alongside opening up breathing pathways.

- Usage: Thyme tea or essential oil (inhalation).

8. **Eucalyptus**

- The plant helps unclog nasal passages while lowering mucus secretion.

- Apply the natural remedy by inhaling or mixing eucalyptus oil with base oils.

Improving Respiratory Health Through Lifestyle

Avoiding Triggers

- Recommendation: Add a list of substances that trigger patients' allergic reactions and teach them how to avoid these items.

Regular Exercise

•	Benefits: Improves lung function and overall respiratory health.

•	Rephrase this section: Moderate-intensity exercises involving walking, swimming, and cycling prove beneficial for therapeutic purposes.

Breathing Exercises

•	Designed breathing exercises enable people to strengthen their breathing muscles and build lung capacity.

•	There are three breathing exercises that provide benefits to lung health: deep breathing exercises, diaphragmatic breathing, and pursed-lip breathing.

Humidifiers

•	Moisture in the air helps minimize respiratory irritation across the space.

•	Usage: Use a humidifier in your home, especially during dry weather or winter months.

Healthy Diet

•	The consumption of this diet supports the health of your respiratory system while minimizing inflammation levels.

•	To support respiratory health, patients should consume nutritious food that combines fruits with vegetables together with whole grains, lean proteins, and healthy fats.

Techniques to Enhance Air Quality at Home

Air Purifiers

•	The use of air purifiers delivers many advantages by drawing allergens and dust along with pollutants out from indoor air.

- High-efficiency particulate air (HEPA) filters should be used to enhance indoor air quality.

Regular Cleaning

- Homeowners who adopt this technique minimize the buildup of airborne allergens along with mold and dust in their environment.

- The recommendation is to vacuum the floor continually and clean surfaces repeatedly along with frequent washing of bedding.

Ventilation

- Room air pollutants decrease while air movements increase when you implement this approach.

- Your home should have open windows and exhaust fans as well as sufficient ventilation.

Natural Cleaning Products

- Your exposure to both chemicals and irritants decreases when you use this product.

- Recommendations: Use natural or non-toxic cleaning products.

Natural Remedies for Specific Respiratory Conditions

Asthma

1. **Herbal Tea**

- Ingredients: Ginger, turmeric, licorice root, honey

- Benefits: Reduces inflammation and soothes the respiratory tract.

- Recipe: Steep ginger, turmeric, and licorice root in hot water for 10 minutes. The mixture requires the addition of desired honey before straining.

2. **Steam Inhalation**

- Ingredients: Eucalyptus oil, hot water

- The use of this remedy opens respiratory pathways and helps minimize respiratory mucus buildup.

- Usage: Add a few drops of eucalyptus oil to hot water. The inhalation steam requires wearing a towel covering your head.

Allergies

1. **Quercetin Supplements**

- Natural antihistamines present in this remedy help decrease allergic reactions.

- Quercetin supplements should be taken according to the provided instructions.

2. **Nettle Tea**

- Benefits: Reduces symptoms of hay fever and allergies.

- Nettle tea should be consumed by you 1-2 times each day.

Chronic Bronchitis

1. **Thyme Tea**

- The antimicrobial attributes present in eucalyptus oil fight respiratory infections at the same time, it reduces congestion.

- Recipe: Steep fresh or dried thyme in hot water for 10 minutes. Strain and drink.

2. **Honey and Lemon**

- The combination of honey with lemon juice in warm water serves two positive health effects: relieving throat pain and controlling coughing.

- Dissolve 1 tablespoon of honey with the juice of one lemon half by mixing them together in warm water.

Sinusitis

1. Neti Pot

- The neti pot provides clearing of nasal passages while decreasing sinus congestion.

- Usage: Use a neti pot with a saline solution to rinse the nasal passages.

2. Steam Inhalation

- Ingredients: Eucalyptus oil, hot water

- Steam treatments through the use of a neti pot lead to opened sinuses while simultaneously easing congestion.

- Usage: Add a few drops of eucalyptus oil to hot water. Cover your head with a towel to steam the mixture with your breath.

Conclusion

Respiratory condition treatment through natural methods requires using herbal medicines together with dietary adjustments and modifications to daily activities. Implementing necessary herbs along with air quality improvements alongside physical activity and breathing exercises helps maintain your respiratory health to effectively deal with regular respiratory conditions. A comprehensive method that emphasizes natural healthcare practices supports long-term respiratory health and overall well-being.

17. Addressing Skin Conditions with Herbs

Natural skin health improvement strategies integrate herbal treatments, dietary adjustments, and safe skincare practices to address conditions such as acne, eczema, and psoriasis. The handbook delivers effective strategies for using herbs when treating prevalent skin problems.

Herbal Treatments for Acne, Eczema, and Psoriasis

Acne

Herbal Remedies

1. **Tea Tree Oil**

• Acne-causing bacteria are reduced effectively by the antimicrobial properties found in these remedies.

• Users should mix the tea tree oil with coconut or jojoba oil before applying it to the skin areas that have acne.

2. **Aloe Vera**

• Tea Tree Oil shows two advantages through its antimicrobial capabilities and soothing properties which minimize redness along with swelling.

• Usage: Apply fresh aloe vera gel directly to the skin.

3. **Witch Hazel**

• This remedy has two advantages because its astringent nature minimizes oil production and tightens skin pores.

• You should apply witch hazel extract on your skin by using a cotton pad.

4. **Green Tea Extract**

•   People who use green tea extract benefit from two key properties that fight acne due to their anti-inflammatory and antioxidant characteristics.

•   Users can benefit from green tea extract applications as well as products infused with this tea.

Eczema

Herbal Remedies

1. **Calendula**

•   The healing effect, combined with the anti-inflammatory properties of this remedy, helps to reduce skin irritation.

•   Usage: Apply calendula cream or oil to affected areas.

2. **Chamomile**

•   The health benefits of green tea extract include its capacity to minimize both itching and skin redness and reduce inflammation.

•   To utilize chamomile remedies for applied relief, you should either apply chamomile-infused oil or cream or make chamomile tea compresses.

3. **Licorice Root**

•   Licorice root extract demonstrates anti-inflammatory properties that minimize eczema conditions.

•   Usage: Apply licorice root extract or cream to the skin.

4. **Oatmeal**

•   Using oatmeal can provide two benefits it soothes dry areas and moisturizes itching skin.

•   People can put colloidal oatmeal in their baths and also benefit from using oatmeal-based creams as a remedy.

Psoriasis

Herbal Remedies

1. Turmeric

• Most psoriasis patients benefit from licorice root because this substance reduces inflammation, which helps manage symptoms.

• The usage of turmeric applications on skin areas with eczema and the consumption of turmeric supplements represent both methods to utilize this remedy.

2. Aloe Vera

• The use of licorice root extract or cream delivers two-fold benefits because it both comforts and hydrates your skin and lowers redness as well as scaling.

• Usage: Apply fresh aloe vera gel directly to the skin.

3. Evening Primrose Oil

• The skin receives two major benefits from using evening primrose oil because it contains essential fatty acids that reduce inflammation and act as a moisturizer.

• The effective method to use evening primrose oil contains topical applications and external consumption through supplements.

4. Oregon Grape

• Patients can benefit from Oregon grape because its antimicrobial and anti-inflammatory makeup promotes psoriasis symptom improvement.

• Usage: Apply Oregon grape extract or cream to the skin.

Diet's Impact on Skin Health

Anti-Inflammatory Diet

1. **Fruits and Vegetables**

• The skin receives essential antioxidants and vitamins through the Oregon grape, which benefits its overall health.

• Examples: Berries, leafy greens, carrots, tomatoes, bell peppers.

2. **Healthy Fats**

• Skin hydration and inflammation reduction are two substantial advantages that essential fatty acids provide to the body.

• Examples: Avocados, nuts, seeds, fatty fish, olive oil.

3. **Whole Grains**

• Eating these foods delivers essential fibers together with vital nutrients that support general health maintenance.

• Examples: Brown rice, quinoa, oats, whole wheat.

4. **Probiotic-Rich Foods**

• Studies show that certain supportive foods benefit gut health as this system affects skin health.

• Examples: Yogurt, kefir, sauerkraut, kimchi, miso.

Foods to Avoid

1. **Sugary Foods**

• The intake of such foods leads to inflammation that worsens skin conditions.

• Examples: Sodas, candies, and pastries.

2. **Processed Foods**

• The health hazards of some skin nutrients occur because processed foods contain unhealthy fats along with problematic additives.

• Natural health foods, which include fast food packaged snacks and refined grains, demonstrate the following issues.

3. **Dairy Products**

• Some users develop skin problems, including acne, because of using dairy products.

• Alternatives: Plant-based milk, lactose-free dairy products.

4. **High Glycemic Index Foods**

• High blood sugar levels may happen when consuming these foods, while inflammation also develops.

• Examples: White bread, white rice, potatoes.

External Applications and Skincare Routines

Natural Skincare Routine

1. **Cleansing**

• The cleansing process takes away oil together with dirt and impurities that reside on the skin's surface.

• Ingredients: Use gentle, natural cleansers like honey or aloe vera.

2. **Exfoliation**

• Dead skin cells get eliminated through this process, which enhances cell turnover.

• Ingredients: Use natural exfoliants like ground oatmeal, sugar, or coffee grounds.

3. **Moisturizing**

• The application of swimming pools with natural moisturizers provides hydration along with skin nourishment benefits.

• Ingredients: Use natural moisturizers like coconut oil, shea butter, or jojoba oil.

4. **Spot Treatments**

• Benefits: Targets specific skin issues like acne or eczema.

• The appropriate treatment ingredients include tea tree oil for acne management alongside calendula cream for eczema.

Herbal Masks

1. **Acne-Prone Skin**

• Ingredients: Honey, turmeric, and yogurt.

• A mixture of one tablespoon of honey and one teaspoon of turmeric combined with one tablespoon of yogurt forms the recipe. After application to the face, allow the mixture to sit for 15-20 minutes then wash it off.

2. **Eczema-Prone Skin**

• Ingredients: Colloidal oatmeal and honey.

• You should mix two tablespoons of colloidal oatmeal with one tablespoon of honey to create this recipe. Mingle the ingredients before applying them to the affected skin, and allow the mixture to stay on for 15 to 20 minutes before you rinse it off.

3. **Psoriasis-Prone Skin**

• Ingredients: Aloe vera gel and turmeric.

• The homemade blend includes two tablespoons of aloe vera gel and one teaspoon of turmeric mixed together. Stir the mixture thoroughly before applying it to the affected skin for 15-20 minutes once, and then wash it off.

Conclusion

Herbal treatment for skin problems requires patients to use therapeutic herbal medicine and make healthy diet changes while following natural skincare practices. You can effectively handle common skin problems by using health-promoting herbs along with nutritious eating and following nature-based skincare practices. A holistic approach emphasizes natural healthcare methods that enhance both short-term and long-term skin health while promoting overall personal wellness.

18. Mental Health and Stress Relief

The preservation of mental health, besides effective stress management, requires attention because it leads to improved overall wellness. A comprehensive approach to mental health combines herbal remedies, lifestyle adjustments, and natural stress relief techniques to promote overall well-being. The guide presents useful methods to support mental health while teaching natural stress management treatments.

Herbs for Mood Improvement and Anxiety Reduction

1. **St. John's Wort**

• The plant proved useful for antidepressant treatment because it manages symptoms of mild to moderate depression along with mood improvement.

• Two applications of St. John's Wort exist as supplements alongside tea.

• You should check with a doctor before using this medicine since it affects numerous drugs with your current medications.

2. **Ashwagandha**

• An adaptogenic agent helps users control their stress response and minimize anxiety symptoms.

• Ashwagandha supplements and powder are available for usage through smoothies or water consumption.

• You should use the dosage listed on the product label but receiving doctor approval remains important.

3. **Valerian Root**

• The herb provides mental relaxation to decrease anxiety symptoms together with better sleep patterns.

- Usage: Valerian root tea, capsules, or tincture.

- The recommended dose of this medication is to take it during night-time hours as a sleep aid.

4. **Lavender**

- The main advantage of using Lavender is its ability to create relaxation effects that control anxiety while boosting mood.

- Usage: Lavender essential oil (aromatherapy), lavender tea.

- People should utilize lavender essential oil through either skin application with diluted drops or by adding the oil to a diffuser.

5. **Lemon Balm**

- Users can receive three advantages from using lemon balm products which include anxiety relief alongside mood elevation and relaxation.

- Usage: Lemon balm tea, capsules, or tincture.

- Use all products according to their indicated dosages shown on labels or seek medical professional advice for recommended amounts.

6. **Passionflower**

- The usage of lavender produces advantages that assist people in managing anxiety and improving their capacity to sleep.

- Usage: Passionflower tea, capsules, or tincture.

- The recommended usage time for this medication is before bedtime to achieve relaxation.

Daily Habits for Mental Wellness

1. **Regular Physical Activity**

- Taking lemon balm products can benefit the mood and reduce anxiety while simultaneously promoting better mental health through endorphin and other pleasure hormone releases.

- Walking, jogging, yoga, and swimming, together with cycling represent recommended physical activities.

- To obtain mental health benefits, take at least 30 minutes of moderate exercise during six or more weekday sessions.

2. Balanced Diet

- A nutritious diet ensures mental wellness because necessary elements fund brain operation and mood stability.

- Healthy food choices consist of whole grains, lean proteins, fruits, vegetables, nuts and seeds, and healthy fats.

- Avoid: Excessive sugar, caffeine, and processed foods.

3. Adequate Sleep

- Benefits: Essential for cognitive function, emotional regulation, and overall well-being.

- To achieve better sleep, people should develop a daily schedule along with calming evening routines while making sure their sleeping space is comfortable.

- It is important to achieve between 7 to 9 hours of high-quality sleep every night.

4. Hydration

- The brain, along with mood, needs proper hydration to function properly.

- Consuming lots of water in small amounts daily, together with hydrating food choices such as fruits and vegetables.

5. Mindfulness and Meditation

- The practice leads to lower stress levels combined with better mental focus while providing strong mental wellness improvements.

- People can use three mindfulness meditation techniques along with guided meditation and deep breathing techniques to practice.

- People should practice mindfulness every day, no matter how brief their sessions may be.

Stress Management and Relaxation Practices

1. **Deep Breathing Exercises**

- Activation of the body's relaxing response enables stress reduction combined with anxiety reduction through these activities.

- You should follow this technique to perform deep breathing by using your nose to inhale for several seconds before holding your breath and mouth to exhale slowly.

2. **Progressive Muscle Relaxation**

- Users can gain two advantages from this method: it reduces bodily tension and releases relaxation over time.

- People should practice muscle tension followed by controlled relaxation, starting with their feet and progressing toward their heads.

3. **Aromatherapy**

- Perfilabs essential oils generate relaxation benefits that help reduce stress levels.

- Oils: Lavender, chamomile, bergamot, ylang-ylang.

- The usage of these essential oils includes adding drops to a diffuser or putting them in bath water and applying diluted skin solutions.

4. **Yoga and Tai Chi**

- People enjoy this practice because it blends both physical exercise and breathing workouts paired with meditation, which results in stress reduction and enhanced mental health.

- Joining a class under professional supervision or viewing online videos online allows the home practice of the chosen techniques.

5. **Journaling**

- Keeping a journal enables people to communicate their feelings through writing while creating a stress management outlet that improves their mental clarity.

- The regular written expression of personal thoughts, experiences, and feelings represents the technique.

6. **Spending Time in Nature**

- The practice leads to improved moods and decreased stress as well as well-rounded betterment of personal wellness.

- The activities involve walking in the park with hiking trips, gardening work and outdoor relaxation.

Enhancing Immune Function

Herbs and Foods

1. **Echinacea**

- Taking Echinacea provides two main advantages which include better immunity and stronger resistance to infections.

- Usage: Echinacea tea, capsules, or tincture.

2. **Elderberry**

- The antioxidant and vitamin constituents in elderberries deliver both benefits to immune system function.

- Usage: Elderberry syrup, gummies, or capsules.

3. **Ginger**

- Ginger demonstrates anti-inflammatory capabilities and functions as an antioxidant to strengthen the immune system.

- The intake of fresh ginger tea comes together with ginger capsules or by adding fresh ginger to food for a beneficial immune system.

4. **Turmeric**

- Black ginger contains anti-inflammatory and antioxidant properties that promote overall health benefits.

- Turmeric tea with capsules and turmeric, in addition to meals, represents valid usage forms.

5. **Vitamin C-rich foods**

- Sources: Citrus fruits, strawberries, bell peppers, broccoli.

- The ingestion of Echinacea provides two advantages: by strengthens immune function while protecting against infections.

Daily Practices

1. **Hydration**

- Assistance from these foods leads to maximal immune system functioning alongside overall health reinforcement.

- The intake of plenty of water is essential together with hydration meals that include various fruits and vegetables.

2. **Regular Exercise**

- Benefits: Improves immune function and overall health.

- People should exercise moderately for at least 30 minutes during seven out of their weekly days.

3. **Adequate Sleep**

- Immune function depends on water consumption because it maintains overall well-being.

- The sleep goal should be to achieve 7-9 hours of excellent sleep during each night.

4. Healthy Diet

• The diet provides essential nutrients that support immune system health functions.

• The recommended foods for immune health include whole grains along with lean proteins, fruits and vegetables, and nuts and seeds with healthy fats.

Conclusion

The path to better mental health alongside stress management includes using natural medications in combination with life adjustments and natural approaches. The combination of useful herbs with proper healthy routines alongside stress-reduction techniques allows you to protect your mental health while decreasing stress levels. The complete mental healthcare system focuses on natural approaches to achieve sustainable mental wellness and general wellness.

19. Enhancing Immune Function

The protection of infections and diseases alongside overall wellness depends on having a robust immune system. Countless scientific reports highlight the effectiveness of comprehensive techniques that enhance immune health by integrating nutritional choices, herbal solutions, and daily wellness activities. The guidance presents natural methods that can help increase immune system strength.

Boosting Immunity with Specific Herbs and Foods

Herbs

1. Echinacea

• Echinacea demonstrates two key functions including immune system support as well as infection-fighting capability.

• Usage: Echinacea tea, capsules, or tincture.

• The product label will guide you on the proper dosage or you should ask for medical advice.

2. Elderberry

• Elderberries provide several antioxidants and vitamins that strengthen immune health.

• Usage: Elderberry syrup, gummies, or capsules.

• The recommended product dosage must be followed as written on the label, or a healthcare provider can recommend an appropriate amount.

3. Ginger

• Immune health receives support from Echinacea through its two key properties, which include anti-inflammatory and antioxidant abilities.

- Users can benefit from ginger tea combined with capsules and raw ginger added to their food for consumption or usage.

- The recommended amount of this supplement is to incorporate it into daily meals or use it as an additional supplement dose.

4. **Turmeric**

- Elderberry syrup and gummies, along with capsules, contain two major benefits, including antioxidant protection and anti-inflammatory benefits, which help support immune health.

- Turmeric tea, along with capsules, represents one usage method along with the option to add this spice to meals, and the recommended dosage should follow the product label or receive medical advice.

- One should add elderberry ingredients to their daily diet or consume it in prescribed supplement forms.

5. **Astragalus**

- An intake of astragalus aids immune function while protecting against infections.

- Usage: Astragalus tea, capsules, or tincture.

- Patients should use the stated recommended dosage found on the product label or get professional medical guidance before taking the drug.

6. **Garlic**

- Benefits: Antimicrobial and immune-boosting properties.

- Usage: Fresh garlic in meals, garlic supplements.

- Daily consumption of macros or supplementing the diet with this product provides the desired health benefits.

Foods

1. Citrus Fruits

• Sources: Oranges, lemons, limes, grapefruits.

• Astragalus provides high levels of vitamin C that strengthens immune defenses.

2. Berries

• Sources: Blueberries, strawberries, raspberries, blackberries.

• The content of antioxidants in these foods helps to strengthen the immune system.

3. Leafy Greens

• Sources: Spinach, kale, Swiss chard.

• The nutritional content includes numerous vitamin and mineral elements that promote total body wellness.

4. Nuts and Seeds

• Sources: Almonds, sunflower seeds, chia seeds, flaxseeds.

• The consumption of these food sources provides beneficial fat along with essential minerals that strengthen the immune response.

5. Yogurt

• The presence of probiotics in this product supports both gut health and strengthens the immune system.

• Usage: Choose yogurt with live and active cultures.

6. Green Tea

• The immune system benefits from antioxidants together with other immune-supporting elements that exist in green tea.

• Usage: Drink green tea daily. Daily Practices for Disease Prevention Hydration

Daily Practices for Disease Prevention

Hydration

- Drinking sufficient water has two important advantages because it supports total body health while maintaining the immune system's peak operation level.

- The recommended serving methods include drinking enough water and including water-rich food such as vegetables and fruits.

Regular Exercise

- The practice of exercise provides benefits at two levels: it enhances immune functions and strengthens overall wellness.

- People should pursue at least 30 minutes of moderate exercise routine for at least six days of the week.

- Persons should perform walking exercises along with jogging exercises, yoga, swimming activities and cycling to improve their health.

Adequate Sleep

- A sufficient amount of sleep is vital for immune functioning and promotes general well-being in the body.

- The sleep goal should be to achieve seven to nine hours of high-quality rest daily.

- To develop a proper sleep routine people should choose a consistent sleep schedule together with stress-free bedtime practices and regulate their sleep environment.

Stress Management

- Exercise helps decrease the way stress influences immune system health.

- Practice relaxation techniques, including meditation, deep breathing exercises, and yoga, along with mindfulness as methods to reduce stress effects on the immune system.

Healthy Diet

- The consumption of essential nutrients through this practice leads to improved immune system health.

- The recommended foods include whole grains and lean proteins together with fruits, vegetables, nuts, seeds, and health-promoting fats.

- Avoid: Excessive sugar, caffeine, and processed foods.

Sunlight Exposure

- The body benefits from vitamin D formation that supports immune function through sunlight exposure.

- Subjects should purposefully spend between 15 and 30 minutes under natural sunlight during daytime.

Sleep's Role in Immune Health

Importance of Sleep

- The proper functioning of the immune system depends on a sufficient amount of sleep each night. The body generates essential components known as cytokines throughout sleep time to combat infections in addition to inflammation.

- Proper sleep duration helps people reduce their stress levels, thus strengthening immunity.

Tips for Better Sleep

1. **Regular Sleep Schedule**

- You should establish consistent bedtime and waking times both during weekdays and on weekends.

- You should create a relaxing framework before bedtime to send sleep signals to your body.

- Your body understands through signals when it reaches the point of preparing for rest.

2.   **Sleep Environment**

•   You need to create a restful sleeping space which should be peaceful and cool while being comfortable.

•   A dark setting in the room helps stimulate the production of melatonin, which functions as the sleep hormone.

3.   **Limit Screen Time**

•   Screen devices like phones and computers with TVs and tablets should be eliminated completely during the hour before sleeping since blue light exposure stops you from resting properly.

4.   **Avoid Stimulants**

•   Your ability to fall asleep becomes impaired when you take caffeine or nicotine within several hours before bed.

Conclusion

A well-functioning immune system emerges from consuming appropriate foods and utilizing medicinal plants along with following healthy living habits. Your immune system, together with your overall health, receives better support when you combine immune-enhancing herbs and proper nutrition with hydration and exercise and adequate sleep and stress management along with outdoor sun exposure. A comprehensive strategy that relies on natural solutions supports sustainable immune health and overall well-being.

20. Women's Health: Natural Approaches

Women's wellness requires dedicated healthcare focusing on hormone management along with reproductive healthcare as well as total personal health support. An approach that combines natural treatments, modified diets, and lifestyle adjustments supports overall well-being and health. This guide presents clear steps to handle menopausal and menstrual symptoms and upgrade reproductive health combined with wellness improvement.

Natural Management of Menstrual and Menopausal Symptoms

Herbal Remedies

1. **Chaste Tree Berry (Vitex)**

•   The use of Chaste Tree Berry produces several advantages that lead to regulated menstrual cycles while decreasing PMS symptoms and managing hormones.

•   Usage: Chaste tree berry supplements or tincture.

•   Follow the suggested dosage instructions provided on the product label while also getting advice from healthcare providers.

2. **Black Cohosh**

•   Benefits: Eases menopausal symptoms such as hot flashes, mood swings, and night sweats.

•   Usage: Black cohosh supplements or tincture.

•   Use the specified dosage instructions provided on the product packaging while also obtaining professional healthcare advice.

3. **Evening Primrose Oil**

- The GLA content in this supplement aids in relieving PMS symptoms as well as menopausal symptoms.

- Usage: Evening primrose oil supplements.

- The dosage instructions should be followed from the product label or you should receive advice from a healthcare professional.

4. **Red Clover**

- This herb contains phytoestrogens, which act as a treatment method for menopausal symptoms.

- Red clover tea and supplements serve as two methods to receive the benefits of this product.

- Patients should use products at the dosages provided on the label or with medical professional advice.

5. **Ginger**

- Benefits: Reduces menstrual pain and inflammation.

- Fresh ginger tea, along with ginger capsules and adding fresh ginger to food, provide the most useful treatments.

- You can include this supplement in your regular meals when having daily dietary consumption.

Dietary Adjustments

1. **Increase Calcium and Magnesium**

- Users can benefit from red clover together with its two key advantages which include pain reduction for menstrual cramps and better bone health support.

- Logan Library contains leafy greens together with almonds and sesame seeds dairy products, and plant-based milk that has additional fortification.

2. **Healthy Fats**

- Benefits: Supports hormonal balance.

- Sources: Avocados, nuts, seeds, olive oil, fatty fish.

3. **Iron-Rich Foods**

- Consuming sufficient amounts of iron aids in preventing conditions of iron deficiency anemia that often occur during a woman's menstrual period.

- Sources: Red meat, poultry, beans, lentils, spinach.

4. **Hydration**

- Drinking water together with consuming water-rich food helps manage bloating while supporting overall health benefits.

- The key sources for staying hydrated include drinking plenty of water together with foods such as cucumbers and watermelon that contain water content.

5. **Whole Grains**

- Benefits: Provides fiber and essential nutrients.

- Sources: Brown rice, quinoa, oats, whole wheat.

Lifestyle Changes

1. **Regular Exercise**

- People who exercise regularly experience reduced PMS symptoms together with better mood and improved overall health.

- Land-based aerobic exercise such as walking, jogging, yoga, swimming, and cycling make up Activities.

- To achieve health benefits you should exercise moderately for a minimum of 30 minutes during at least thirty days per week.

2. **Stress Management**

- Benefits: Reduces the impact of stress on hormonal balance and overall health.

- The practice of meditation combined with deep breathing along with yoga and mindfulness constitute relaxation techniques that help create balance.

3. **Adequate Sleep**

- Benefits: Essential for overall health and hormonal balance.

- People should achieve trouble-free sleep with a duration of 7 to 9 hours throughout each night.

- People should establish a steady sleep pattern and develop calming nighttime routines as well as maintain the comfort of their sleep space.

Herbs for Hormonal Balance and Reproductive Health

Herbal Remedies

1. **Maca Root**

- Hormonal balance, together with better fertility, constitute the benefits of this remedy.

- Usage: Maca powder or capsules.

- People should follow either the dosage instructions mentioned on product labels or seek medical professional advice.

2. **Ashwagandha**

- The consumption of Ashwagandha minimizes stress while helping maintain hormonal stability in the body.

- Ashwagandha supplements, as well as powder, are available through smoothies or water for consumption.

• It is necessary to use the dosage levels specified on the product label or seek professional medical advice from a healthcare provider.

3. **Shatavari**

• Benefits: Supports reproductive health and hormonal balance.

• Usage: Shatavari powder or capsules.

• The recommended dosage of the product appears on its label, or a healthcare provider can provide specific guidance.

4. **Dong Quai**

• The substance delivers positive benefits for blood circulation and menstrual health regulations.

• Dong Quai supplements and tinctures serve as proper ways of usage.

• The product label contains recommended dosage instructions, or people should receive healthcare professional advice on appropriate amounts.

Fertility Enhancement Through Natural Means

Nutritional Support

1. **Folate**

• Benefits: Essential for healthy fetal development.

• People should consume leafy greens, beans, and lentils, along with citrus fruits and fortified cereals.

2. **Zinc**

• Benefits: Supports reproductive health and hormone production.

• Sources: Meat, shellfish, nuts, seeds, dairy products.

3. **Vitamin D**

•   The consumption of these nutrients provides benefits for reproductive wellness together with whole-body well-being.

•   The primary sources to obtain these components include sunlight exposure and, fatty fish items and fortified foods or supplements.

4. **Omega-3 Fatty Acids**

•   Benefits: Supports hormonal balance and overall health.

•   Sources: Fatty fish, flaxseeds, chia seeds, walnuts.

Lifestyle Changes

1. **Maintain a Healthy Weight**

•   Benefits: Supports hormonal balance and reproductive health.

•   People should merge eating nutritious food with exercising physical activities.

2. **Avoid Alcohol and Smoking**

•   Regular exercise combined with the avoidance of alcohol and smoking reduces infertility risk while also improving general health.

•   People should refrain from alcohol and smoking, but they can also find assistance to stop using these substances.

3. **Regular Exercise**

•   Exercise as a health benefit promotes total well-being and minimizes stress levels.

•   Walking, jogging along with yoga, swimming, cycling, and yoga comprise the recommended physical exercises.

•   A person must perform 30 minutes of moderate exercise activities for at least five days during each week.

4.   **Stress Management**

•   Benefits: Reduces the impact of stress on fertility and overall health.

•   Practicing meditation and deep breathing exercises, as well as yoga and mindfulness, represents the techniques for managing stress.

Conclusion

The natural support of women's health requires a full assessment through herbal medicine, dietary improvements, and modified lifestyle patterns. Your effective well-being support will result from following natural approaches that help manage menstrual symptoms and menopause symptoms and improve reproductive health and overall wellness. A holistic approach emphasizes natural healthcare methods to support women's long-term well-being.

21. Combating Chronic Inflammation

Different health problems, such as heart disease, diabetes, arthritis, and specific forms of cancer, develop from persistent inflammation. A comprehensive approach to reducing inflammation includes carefully selected foods, lifestyle adjustments, and natural treatment options. The guide contains real-world methods that help people fight chronic inflammation beneficially.

Anti-Inflammatory Diet and Lifestyle Adjustments

Anti-Inflammatory Foods

1. **Fruits and Vegetables**

- Eating such foods delivers antioxidants along with vitamins and minerals, which help decrease inflammation in the body.

- Examples: Berries (blueberries, strawberries, raspberries), leafy greens (spinach, kale, Swiss chard), tomatoes, bell peppers, carrots, broccoli.

2. **Healthy Fats**

- Foods containing omega-3 essential fatty acids provide strong anti-inflammatory abilities to the body.

- Foods that benefit inflammation include the following:(State the points explicitly. Also normalize verbalization when possible)

3. **Whole Grains**

- Whole grains offer two major benefits by delivering fiber, which helps both health and reduces inflammation together with essential nutrients.

- Sources: Brown rice, quinoa, oats, whole wheat, barley.

4. **Herbs and Spices**

• The human body benefits from the consumption of these foods because they contain anti-inflammatory compounds that promote overall health.

• Examples: Turmeric, ginger, garlic, cinnamon, rosemary, thyme.

5. **Probiotic-Rich Foods**

• Gut health benefits present through these foods lead to reduced inflammation.

• Sources: Yogurt, kefir, sauerkraut, kimchi, miso.

6. **Green Tea**

• Green tea includes antioxidants that fight inflammation and benefit health in both ways.

• Usage: Drink green tea daily.

Foods to Avoid

1. **Processed Foods**

• These foods contain unhealthful fats, together with excessive sugars and additives, which can trigger inflammatory responses in the body.

• Fast food, together with packaged snacks and sugary cereals, make up examples of foods to avoid in the diet.

2. **Refined Carbohydrates**

• A typical high-sugar intake leads to blood sugar spikes at the same time, it raises the amount of inflammation in the body.

• Examples: White bread, white rice, and pastries.

3. **Sugary Foods and Beverages**

• Consistent high consumption of sugar creates increased body inflammation.

• Certain examples of these harmful items include sodas, candies, pastries, and sweetened beverages.

4. **Trans Fats**

• Various health conditions arise because trans fats both increase inflammation and create different health problems.

• The main food sources of trans fats include both fried items and margarine, together with processed bakery products.

5. **Excessive Alcohol**

• Too much ingestion of these foods leads to increased inflammation which simultaneously affects our overall health condition for the worse.

• It is essential to minimize alcohol consumption up to total avoidance of alcohol.

Lifestyle Adjustments

1. **Regular Physical Activity**

• Regular exercise offers multiple advantages by lowering inflammation and enhancing cardiovascular operations together with enhancing overall wellness.

• Walking alongside jogging, together with swimming, yoga, and cycling, serve as acceptable activities.

• People should exercise moderately at least thirty minutes daily with a minimum of six sessions each week.

2. **Stress Management**

• Benefits: Reduces the impact of stress on inflammation and overall health.

• Individuals should practice deep breathing exercises alongside meditation along with yoga and mindfulness as relaxation techniques.

3. **Adequate Sleep**

• Getting sufficient rest serves as an essential anti-inflammatory method that promotes general health benefits.

• Set the target of achieving 7-9 hours of quality sleeping duration each night.

• People should establish daily sleep patterns and develop calming night routines while maintaining appropriate sleeping conditions.

4. **Hydration**

Hospital personnel who maintain proper hydration receive health advantages while minimizing inflammatory responses.

Water intake should be constant throughout the day, along with eating hydrating foods like fruits together with vegetables.

Herbal Anti-Inflammatories and Their Usage

1. **Turmeric**

• Benefits: Contains curcumin, a potent anti-inflammatory compound.

• The use of turmeric tea alongside capsules and the inclusion of turmeric in cooked dishes constitutes its recommended applications.

• The necessary amount of each substance can be found on product labels, or patients should seek advice from healthcare providers.

2. Ginger

• Turmeric provides anti-inflammatory properties while simultaneously benefiting a person's overall health condition.

• Fresh ginger tea and ginger capsules together with fresh ginger in prepared meals serve as usage methods for this anti-inflammatory remedy.

• Testing your body requires daily consumption of meals containing turmeric and supplements or simple use of turmeric supplements.

3. Boswellia

• This substance brings two advantages to the table: minimizing inflammation and maintaining joint health.

• Usage: Boswellia supplements or extract.

• You should use the dosage from the product label or get professional medical advice.

4. Green Tea Extract

• The antioxidants in this remedy work to decrease inflammation inside the body.

• Usage: Green tea or green tea extract supplements.

• The recommended dosage of green tea consists of daily consumption through drinking or supplement usage.

5. Willow Bark

• The main advantage of willow bark extract is its salicin content which works as an anti-inflammatory component.

• Usage: Willow bark tea, capsules, or tincture.

• The dosage instructions should match those mentioned on the product label, while healthcare provider advice remains an option.

Understanding Inflammation's Role in Chronic Diseases

Impact of Chronic Inflammation

1. **Cardiovascular Diseases**

•	Chronic inflammation causes atherosclerosis to develop, which subsequently raises the risk factors for heart attacks together with strokes.

•	Prevention: Maintain a healthy diet, regular physical activity, and stress management.

2. **Diabetes**

•	The inflammatory process disrupts the way insulin signals work, thus causing insulin resistance and type 2 diabetes.

•	To prevent chronic inflammation people should consume an anti-inflammatory diet alongside exercising regularly and keeping their body weight in check.

3. **Arthritis**

•	The presence of inflammation in joints produces painful stiffness which appears among rheumatoid arthritis and osteoarthritis patients.

•	People should prevent diabetes onset and arthritis development by maintaining their weight and engaging in active exercise alongside the use of anti-inflammatory foods and herbs.

4. **Cancer**

•	The development, together with the progression of specific cancers, can happen because of persistent inflammatory states.

•	Anti-inflammatory nutrition should be combined with healthy life choices, along with medicinal plants and anti-inflammatory foods for prevention purposes.

5. **Neurodegenerative Diseases**

- Because inflammation exists within the brain, it plays a role in diseases like Alzheimer's and Parkinson's.

- Apart from following a healthy diet with abundant antioxidants one needs to stay active while controlling their stress levels.

Conclusion

The treatment of chronic inflammation requires a three-step method which involves following an anti-inflammatory diet together with changing lifestyle habits and using natural herbal remedies. You can support both your health and decrease inflammation through the combination of anti-inflammatory food intake along with physical activity and stress management, adequate sleep, and confirmed use of beneficial herbs. Holistic practices emphasize natural approaches to achieving sustainable health benefits.

22. Cancer Prevention and Support

Modern cancer prevention focuses on the combination of proper nutrition and lifestyle changes together with natural healing approaches, which assist both prevention and current patient care. A comprehensive cancer prevention system supports health on multiple levels through balanced nutrition, lifestyle adjustments, and natural wellness practices. A guide offering useful cancer prevention methods and supportive treatment strategies is delivered.

A Holistic Approach to Cancer Prevention

Key Principles

1. **Healthy Diet**

- Focus on whole, unprocessed foods.

- A healthy diet requires a combination of different fruits, veggies, complete grains, lean proteins, and nutritious fats.

- People should eliminate processed foods as well as sugary snacks and both red and processed meats must be avoided in limited quantities.

2. **Regular Physical Activity**

- Aim for at least 150 minutes of moderate-intensity exercise per week.

- The fitness plan should contain two exercise categories including aerobic workouts (such as walking, jogging, swimming) and strength training activities.

3. **Maintaining a Healthy Weight**

- Balance caloric intake with physical activity.

- People should maintain a lean weight while trying to achieve their target BMI.

4. **Avoiding Tobacco**

- Smoking, along with secondhand smoke exposure, should be completely avoided.

- The individual should seek assistance to stop smoking in case they are currently smoking.

5. **Limiting Alcohol Consumption**

- Limit alcohol intake to one drink per day for women and two drinks per day for men.

6. **Sun Protection**

- Individuals should apply sunscreen, dress properly, and avoid overexposure to the sun in order to decrease their risk of skin cancer.

7. **Regular Health Screenings**

- Participate in regular screenings for early detection of cancer, such as mammograms, colonoscopies, and Pap smears.

Nutritional Guidelines for Cancer Prevention

Anti-Cancer Foods

1. **Cruciferous Vegetables**

- These vegetables contain sulforaphane compounds, which research shows lower the danger of cancer development.

- Examples: Broccoli, cauliflower, Brussels sprouts, kale.

2. **Berries**

- The antioxidants present in this food act as cellular protectors against damage.

- Examples: Blueberries, strawberries, raspberries, blackberries.

3. **Leafy Greens**

- Benefits: Rich in vitamins, minerals, and fiber that support overall health.

- Examples: Spinach, kale, Swiss chard, and arugula.

4. **Tomatoes**

- The cancer-preventing compound lycopene exists within tomatoes and research shows it decreases the risk of prostate cancer along with other cancers.

- The diet benefits from incorporating both fresh and cooked tomatoes and tomato sauces along with other tomato-based foods.

5. **Garlic**

- Research indicates that the compounds present in these foods fight against cancer development.

- Regular meals benefit from fresh garlic addition or garlic supplements provide a similar benefit.

6. **Green Tea**

- The antioxidants alongside polyphenols in this food group support human health while lowering cancer risks.

- Usage: Drink green tea daily.

7. **Turmeric**

- Benefits: Contains curcumin, which has anti-inflammatory and anti-cancer properties.

- Usage: Add turmeric to meals or take turmeric supplements.

Foods to Avoid

1. **Processed Meats**

- Issues: Linked to an increased risk of colorectal cancer.

- Examples: Sausages, hot dogs, bacon.

2. **Sugary Foods and Beverages**

- High amounts of sugar create obesity risks, which provide conditions for multiple kinds of cancer formation.

- Examples: Sodas, candies, and pastries.

3. **Refined Carbohydrates**

- The consumption of these food items triggers sudden blood sugar elevation and generates inflammatory processes.

- Examples: White bread, white rice, and pastries.

4. **Excessive Alcohol**

- Issues: Increases the risk of cancers, particularly of the mouth, throat, esophagus, liver, breast, and colon.

- The recommendation is to refrain from alcohol or to limit alcohol use to the lowest possible amount.

Supportive Herbs for Cancer Prevention and Support

Herbal Remedies

1. **Green Tea Extract**

- The antioxidant polyphenols, together with anti-inflammatory antioxidants in these plants, promote overall health benefits.

- Consuming green tea through daily consumption or taking extract supplements constitutes a proper usage approach.

2. **Turmeric (Curcumin)**

- Benefits: Anti-inflammatory and anti-cancer properties.

- Usage: Add turmeric to meals or take curcumin supplements.

3. **Milk Thistle**

•	Benefits: Supports liver health and detoxification.

•	Usage: Milk thistle tea, capsules, or tincture.

4. **Ginger**

•	The usage of this ingredient brings both inflammation reduction and general health promotion benefits.

•	The three possible applications of fresh ginger as a medicine include drinking ginger tea, taking ginger capsules, and consuming fresh ginger as part of meals.

5. **Astragalus**

•	Benefits: Supports immune function and overall health.

•	Usage: Astragalus tea, capsules, or tincture.

Integrating Natural Care with Conventional Treatments

Working with Healthcare Providers

1. **Consult with Professionals**

•	Consult with your healthcare provider regarding natural remedies as well as supplements since they may affect your conventional medical treatment.

2. **Complementary Therapies**

•	Use natural remedies as complementary therapies alongside conventional treatments for holistic care.

3. **Personalized Plans**

•	Create a custom-made healthcare plan that contains diet adjustments combined with herbal medicines and lifestyle adaptations based on your personal requirements.

Supporting Overall Well-being

1.   Stress Management

•   The use of stress reduction methods produces two advantages: it protects general health and strengthens the immune response. The methods include practicing meditation along with deep breathing exercises and yoga and mindfulness as your personal relaxation techniques.

2.   Regular Exercise

•   Physical exercise provides multiple advantages through supporting health stress reduction and mood improvement. People who choose this plan should engage in walking, jogging, yoga, swimming, and cycling as their physical exercises. Exercise consumption must reach at least 30 minutes of moderate intensity for at least four days throughout the week.

3.   Adequate Sleep

•   Benefits: Essential for overall health and recovery.

•   The goal should be to obtain 7-9 hours of nightly quality sleep.

•   Successful sleep requires people to follow a steady sleep pattern while using calming bedtime practices within comfortable sleeping conditions.

Conclusion

Preventing cancer alongside supporting total health requires a complete program, which includes choosing diet foods alongside adjusting lifestyle measures and using natural treatment options. Your cancer risk reduction, together with strengthened health outcomes, depends on your consumption of anti-cancer foods along with physical movement and stress regulation, sufficient rest, and the incorporation of health-supporting herbs. Natural prevention methods serve as a key path to achieving sustainable health benefits and long-term cancer prevention through mindful nutrition, lifestyle choices, and holistic wellness practices.

23. Easing Migraines and Headaches

The presence of migraines, together with headaches, distorts regular activities in addition to causing persistent physical challenges. A comprehensive approach to managing and alleviating medical conditions involves selecting specific foods, implementing lifestyle adjustments, and utilizing natural remedies. Readers will find concrete methods in this guide that help prevent and reduce suffering from migraines along with headaches.

Identifying Triggers and Natural Preventative Measures

Common Triggers

1. **Stress**

- The practice of meditation, together with deep breathing exercises and yoga, forms part of the stress management plan.

2. **Dietary Factors**

- Various diet items that can trigger symptoms include caffeine, alcohol, aged cheeses, processed foods, artificial sweeteners, and food additives.

- A food diary will help identify food triggers, which you must record to prevent their consumption.

3. **Sleep Disturbances**

- A regular sleep schedule with proper sleep quality both play essential roles in management.

4. **Dehydration**

- You should drink plenty of water as a prevention measure throughout each day.

5.   **Hormonal Changes**

•   Physicians should track hormonal changes to manage them by adjusting both dietary and lifestyle activities.

6.   **Environmental Factors**

•   The most typical events that trigger symptoms include bright lights in combination with loud noises and strong smells.

•   To manage these issues, individuals should utilize earplugs together with sunglasses to reduce their exposure to pungent odors.

Effective Herbal Remedies and Dosages

Herbal Remedies

1.   **Feverfew**

•   Benefits: Reduces the frequency and severity of migraines.

•   Usage: Feverfew tea, capsules, or tincture.

•   The dosage instructions should be followed either by checking product labels or seeking advice from a healthcare professional.

2.   **Butterbur**

•   Benefits: Reduces the frequency of migraine attacks.

•   Usage: Butterbur supplements (PA-free).

•   Relief seekers should follow both the package labeling dosage and seek professional healthcare advice to establish proper usage amounts.

3.   **Ginger**

•   The consumption of ginger provides two main advantages by reducing both headache-related pain and inflammation.

•   Fresh ginger tea provides benefits when accompanied by ginger capsules and the addition of fresh ginger to eating meals.

- One should include this supplement in their daily food intake or take it as a separate medication.

4. Peppermint Oil

- The application of peppermint oil provides cooling effects and helps to cut down headache symptoms.

- Peppermint oil should be applied in a diluted amount to the area around your forehead and temples.

- The recommended usage is to apply this substance when needed for treating headaches.

5. Lavender Oil

- Using peppermint oil in this manner offers relaxation while easing headache symptoms.

- The 4 usage methods for lavender oil include the use of the diffuser system and application on the temples using diluted solution and lung inhalation methods.

- The recommended dose of this remedy is to use it whenever you need headache relief.

Lifestyle Adjustments for Migraine Sufferers

Regular Physical Activity

- The use of this remedy enhances people's general wellness along with their stress management and prevents migraine attacks.

- Walking together with jogging serves as well as yoga practice alongside swimming and cycling exercises as part of regular activities.

- Make moderate exercise part of your routine by allocating 30 minutes for active sessions every day except for two.

Healthy Diet

- Anti-Inflammatory Foods: Incorporate foods rich in omega-3 fatty acids, antioxidants, and vitamins.

- Examples: Fatty fish, leafy greens, berries, nuts, seeds, and olive oil.

- Find and eliminate all dietary components that produce migraines.

- Warms up your body with a lot of water during the day because dehydration leads to migraine attacks.

Stress Management

- Exercises in relaxation methods, including meditation and deep breathing, together with yoga and mindfulness practices, should be practiced.

- Develop a regular schedule that includes stress management techniques for daily practice.

Adequate Sleep

- The prevention of migraines depends on achieving regular sleep of high quality for each night.

- Your sleep schedule must remain consistent in addition to a calming preparation before bedtime combined with an inviting sleeping environment.

- You should invest 7-9 hours daily into achieving high-quality nighttime rest.

Regular Meals

- Your blood sugar stability depends on eating scheduled balanced meals, which helps prevent spikes in blood sugar levels.

- The strategy includes never skipping a meal while consuming foods rich in nutrients.

Monitoring and Managing Triggers

- Record your daily food intake through a diary, as this will help you identify which foods trigger migraines.

- People should use a Migraine Journal to monitor headaches while identifying relationship patterns between head pain and their environment, food choices, and lifestyle choices.

Conclusion

Coping with headaches and migraines demands a thorough methodology, which includes observation of triggers alongside adding herbal treatments, performing lifestyle changes, and sustaining good health. Working together with preventive care and natural treatments and developing healthy life choices will help decrease both the number of migraine attacks along their overall intensity. Natural healthcare methods support sustained health outcomes by addressing migraines and headaches through dietary choices, lifestyle adjustments, and holistic remedies.

24. Natural Remedies for the Common Cold and Flu

To handle common colds and flu, patients must tackle their symptoms while strengthening their immune response and recovering from illness. Treating the cold and flu involves a comprehensive approach that includes specific foods, natural plant compounds, and lifestyle adjustments to support recovery and overall well-being. The guideline contains actionable steps that help people treat the common cold and flu through natural methods.

Immune-Boosting Herbs and Their Preparations

1. Echinacea

•	A strong immunity forms when Echinacea fights viral infections.

•	Usage: Echinacea tea, capsules, or tincture.

•	Preparation: Steep 1 teaspoon of dried echinacea in a cup of hot water for 10 minutes. Drink 2-3 times a day.

2. Elderberry

•	These ingredients in Echinacea contain numerous antioxidants and vitamins that strengthen immune functions.

•	Usage: Elderberry syrup, gummies, or capsules.

•	Daily consumption of elderberry syrup should include one to two teaspoons and should never exceed the product label recommendations.

3. Ginger

•	Using echinacea brings the dual advantage of decreasing inflammation while providing comfort to respiratory tissues.

- People can use fresh ginger tea along with ginger capsules together with fresh ginger as an ingredient in their meals for its health benefits.

- Preparation: Steep a few slices of fresh ginger in a cup of hot water for 10 minutes. However, additional benefits can be gained by mixing honey with lemon. Drink 2-3 times a day.

4. **Garlic**

- Benefits: Antimicrobial and immune-boosting properties.

- Usage: Fresh garlic in meals or garlic supplements.

- Before use, you must crush a clove of garlic and let it rest for ten minutes to activate its beneficial compounds. Eating garlic in its raw form with honey or placing it into meals provides its benefits.

5. **Peppermint**

- The throat receives calming relief, while congestion gets better through the use of this remedy.

- Usage: Peppermint tea or essential oil (inhalation).

- A mixture of 1 teaspoon of dried peppermint leaves in hot water for 10 minutes creates preparation for peppermint tea. Drink 2-3 times a day.

6. **Licorice Root**

- Benefits: Soothes the respiratory tract and reduces inflammation.

- Usage: Licorice root tea or capsules.

- Preparation: Steep 1 teaspoon of dried licorice root in a cup of hot water for 10 minutes. Drink 2-3 times a day.

7. **Thyme**

- The antimicrobial characteristics of this substance fight respiratory infections.

- Usage: Thyme tea or essential oil (inhalation).

- Preparation: Steep 1 teaspoon of dried thyme in a cup of hot water for 10 minutes. Drink 2-3 times a day.

Supportive Dietary Practices During Illness

Hydrating Foods and Beverages

1. **Water**

- Drinking water provides the body with essential water and toxic waste elimination capabilities.

- You should consume ample water amounts all day to stay hydrated.

2. **Herbal Teas**

- Hydration benefits exist alongside additional health advantages that come from these substances.

- Examples: Ginger tea, peppermint tea, chamomile tea.

3. **Broths and Soups**

- The consumption of these foods provides essential hydration together with essential nutrients, and their digestion is easy for the body.

- Examples: Chicken broth vegetable soup.

4. **Citrus Fruits**

- The average portion of citrus fruits contains high levels of vitamin C, which helps patients boost their immune function.

- Examples: Oranges, lemons, grapefruits.

5. **Berries**

- Benefits: Rich in antioxidants and vitamins.

- Examples: Blueberries, strawberries, raspberries.

Nutrient-Rich Foods

1. **Leafy Greens**

• Benefits: Provide vitamins, minerals, and antioxidants.

• Examples: Spinach, kale, Swiss chard.

2. **Garlic and Onions**

• The absorption of compounds through these foods aids the immune system while fighting off infections.

• Usage: Add to soups, stews, and other meals.

3. **Ginger and Turmeric**

• Benefits: Anti-inflammatory and immune-boosting properties.

• Usage: Add to teas, soups, and meals.

4. **Honey**

• Consuming honey provides soothing effects to the throat while also fighting microbial infection.

• Mechanism of Use: People can either dissolve honey in their teas or drink it alone.

5. **Yogurt**

• The consumption of yogurt delivers both probiotics which maintain gut health as well as support immune system function.

• Usage: Include in meals or as a snack.

Hydration and Rest Strategies for Recovery

The Importance of Hydration

1. **Water**

• Drinking water protects hydration and detoxifies the body by removing harmful substances.

- People should consume no less than eight water cups each day.

2. **Electrolyte Solutions**

- The consumption of electrolyte solutions helps replace minerals that escape during sickness.

- Coconut water, together with homemade electrolyte drinks that mix water with salt and lemon, constitute examples of safe replacement solutions.

3. **Herbal Teas**

- Drinking these solutions has two main effects: they hydrate the body and also serve as soothing agents.

- Examples: Chamomile tea, ginger tea, peppermint tea.

Importance of Rest

1. **Adequate Sleep**

- Benefits: Essential for recovery and immune function.

- People should aim to sleep for 7-9 hours of quality sleep during each night.

2. **Rest Periods**

- The body requires this time to mend itself and achieve recovery.

- You should take scheduled napping and resting times during your daily schedule.

3. **Comfortable Environment**

- Benefits: Promotes relaxation and recovery.

- Tips: Create a quiet, dark, and comfortable sleeping environment.

Additional Supportive Practices

1. Humidifiers

- Using humidifiers provides two benefits which include moisture addition to the air together with respiratory relief.

- Usage: Use a humidifier in your room, especially during dry weather or winter months.

2. Steam Inhalation

- The practice of steam inhalation functions to reduce sinus congestion while clearing nasal passages.

- The technique involves using steam inhalation through hot water contained in a bowl while you cover your head with a towel.

3. Saltwater Gargle

- A saltwater gargle relaxes throat pain while also diminishing throat bacterial count.

- Preparation: Mix 1/2 teaspoon of salt in a cup of warm water and gargle several times a day.

4. Nasal Irrigation

- Similar benefits include nasal passage clearing combined with congestion reduction.

- Technique: Use a neti pot with a saline solution.

Conclusion

You can successfully cope with common colds and flu through a complete method that utilizes immune-enhancing herbs with nutritious diets in combination with hydration and sufficient sleep. Using dietary and natural remedies alongside lifestyle practices helps reduce your symptoms along with strengthening your immune system to encourage better healing. A natural approach to health focuses on achieving lasting well-being through balanced nutrition, lifestyle adjustments, and holistic wellness practices.

25. Men's Health: Prostate Support and Vitality

Wellbeing for men depends heavily on both prostate health and maintaining vitality. A comprehensive health strategy combines mindful food selections, plant-based remedies, and lifestyle adjustments to support prostate wellness and enhance energy levels. The guide offers actionable steps that help people protect their prostate while improving their complete vitality in an all-natural way.

Enhancing Men's Health and Vitality

Dietary Recommendations

1. **Increase Fruits and Vegetables**

- These fruits offer multiple benefits because of their antioxidant properties; vitamin content and mineral content that helps build overall health effectively.

- Examples: Berries, tomatoes, leafy greens, cruciferous vegetables (broccoli, cauliflower, Brussels sprouts).

2. **Healthy Fats**

- Benefits: Essential for hormone production and overall health.

- Sources: Avocados, nuts, seeds, olive oil, fatty fish (salmon, mackerel).

3. **Whole Grains**

- Benefits: Provide fiber and essential nutrients.

- Sources: Brown rice, quinoa, oats, whole wheat.

4. **Lean Proteins**

- Benefits: Supports muscle maintenance and overall health.

- Synonymous foods include chicken, turkey, fish, and legumes, as well as tofu eggs alongside turkey and fish.

5. **Antioxidant-Rich Foods**

- One benefit of antioxidant foods includes defense against cellular breakdown and improved prostate health.

- Sources: Berries, dark chocolate, green tea, nuts.

6. **Hydration**

- Benefits: Essential for overall health and detoxification.

- Sources: Water, herbal teas, hydrating fruits and vegetables.

Foods to Avoid

1. **Processed Foods**

- Issues: Often high in unhealthy fats, sugars, and additives.

- Fast food, alongside packaged snacks, also contains sugary cereals, which should be restricted from consumption.

2. **Red and Processed Meats**

- Issues: Linked to an increased risk of prostate cancer.

- People should substitute their meat consumption with lean meats alongside poultry, fish, along plant-based proteins.

3. **Excessive Alcohol**

- These foods present multiple problems that damage the body's health system and raise swelling levels.

- Patients should restrict themselves to non-alcohol consumption.

4. **Sugary Foods and Beverages**

- Issues: Can lead to weight gain and increase inflammation.

- Examples: Sodas, candies, and pastries.

Herbs Specifically Beneficial for Men's Health

Herbal Remedies

1. **Saw Palmetto**

- Saw palmetto provides prostate health benefits that help alleviate benign prostatic hyperplasia (BPH) symptoms.

- Usage: Saw palmetto supplements or tincture.

- The product label should provide the correct dosage amounts, which users should follow, or they can seek medical advice.

2. **Pygeum**

- The ingestion of Saw Palmetto leads to two key health results which are symptom relief of BPH and improved prostate function.

- Usage: Pygeum supplements or tincture.

- You should take the medicine following the dosage advice listed on the product label while also seeking professional healthcare advice.

3. **Stinging Nettle**

- The intake of stinging nettle provides beneficial effects on urinary wellness and symptom relief for BPH patients.

- Usage: Stinging nettle tea, capsules, or tincture.

- Users should follow both label-directed care and seek healthcare professional guidance regarding the proper dosage form.

4. **Pumpkin Seed**

- The plant extract supports prostate health through its effectiveness against urinary symptoms.

- Raw pumpkin seeds are safe for consumption, and pumpkin seed oil supplements should also be taken according to package instructions.

• People should add this substance to their daily food consumption or follow the instructions on product labels for appropriate usage amounts.

5. **Lycopene**

• An antioxidant within lycopene supports prostate health systems naturally.

• Sources: Tomatoes, watermelon, pink grapefruit.

• The consumption of both lycopene-rich foods together with supplements represents a recommended strategy.

6. **Zinc**

• Benefits: Supports prostate health and overall vitality.

• Sources: Meat, shellfish, nuts, seeds, dairy products.

• The addition of zinc-rich foods to your meals or supplementation with zinc represents an excellent option.

Exercise and Stress Reduction for Overall Vitality

1. **Regular Physical Activity**

• Physical exercise benefits the heart while helping muscles stay strong along with lowering stress levels, which lead to better overall vital health.

• The recommended exercises include walking and jogging alongside yoga practice and swimming together with cycling and weight-based workouts.

• The exercise plan must have at least 150 minutes of weekly moderate-intensity workouts that combine aerobic activities with muscle-strengthening exercises.

2. **Stress Management**

- Regular practice creates beneficial health effects that protect the body by reducing stress-related damage as it benefits mental wellness.

- The techniques of meditation and deep breathing exercises combined with yoga practice and making use of mindfulness can help achieve relaxation.

3. **Adequate Sleep**

- Benefits: Essential for overall health, hormone regulation, and recovery.

- Everyone should aim for seven to nine hours of quality sleep each night.

- You should create a fixed sleep schedule while preparing relaxing bedtime activities and organizing a comfortable sleeping space.

4. **Healthy Weight Management**

- Benefits: Reduces the risk of chronic diseases and supports overall vitality.

- People should maintain their weight with a proper combination of eating healthfully and exercising regularly to attain and sustain a fit body.

5. **Hydration**

- Benefits: Essential for overall health and detoxification.

- The daily intake of water should be high, with water-rich fruits and vegetables making up parts of your diet.

Additional Supportive Practices

1. Regular Health Screenings

• The identification of health problems during their early stages proves essential because early intervention permits better treatment of prostate conditions and other medical issues.

• Regular visits to your healthcare provider for screenings should be scheduled as a recommendation.

2. Sunlight Exposure

• Sunlight exposure through short daily periods enables the body to produce vitamin D so humans can maintain excellent health.

• Tips: Spend time outdoors in natural sunlight for at least 15-30 minutes a day.

3. Balanced Lifestyle

• The adoption of this practice supports the preservation of general health in addition to well-being.

• The recommended strategies include balancing your life with nutritional diets combined with physical exercise, proper stress management techniques, and sufficient rest periods.

Conclusion

A man's support for prostate health while successfully managing his vitality includes using dietary choices together with herbal remedies combined with regular physical activity and practicable stress management techniques. Through having a diet with balanced nutrition in fruits and vegetables along with healthy fats, lean proteins, and whole grains combined with beneficial herbs, an active lifestyle, stress minimization, and sufficient sleep, men can protect their prostate health while improving their life vitality. A holistic framework emphasizes natural care methods as the optimal approach for achieving sustainable health benefits in men.

26. Allergy Relief and Management

People who want to control their allergies need to pinpoint their triggers, apply natural care methods, and adopt life-changing behaviors for successful allergy management. Effective allergy relief and management require a comprehensive approach that addresses multiple aspects of health and well-being. Practical strategies within this document teach people how to reduce allergic reactions and enhance their general health state.

Identifying Allergens and Reducing Exposure

Common Allergens

1. Pollen

- Sources: Trees, grasses, weeds.

- The management steps include following pollen forecast reports and keeping windows shut when pollen counts rise along with operating air purifiers.

2. Dust Mites

- Sources: Bedding, carpets, upholstered furniture.

- To control dust mites, individuals should put allergen-proof covers on their beds and do weekly hot-water bed washing while vacuuming their space with a HEPA filter unit.

3. Pet Dander

- Skin flakes, together with saliva and urine from animals, are the sources of this allergen.

- Pet owners should prevent animals from sleeping in the bedroom space, and they should consistently bathe their pets while running indoor air cleaners.

4. **Mold**

•   The main moist environments that create mold growth include kitchens, bathrooms, and basements.

•   Managers should handle mold problems by fixing leaks and cleaning moldy surfaces with vinegar or other natural cleaning agents also involving dehumidifier usage.

5. **Food Allergens**

•   Common Triggers: Peanuts, tree nuts, shellfish, dairy, wheat, soy, eggs.

•   Persons facing allergies must identify their trigger foods through label reading and seek medical help from an allergist to get proper testing.

Herbal Remedies for Allergy Symptoms

1. **Butterbur**

•   This remedy provides two advantages since it both prevents inflammation and controls muscle spasms, which helps people alleviate allergy symptoms.

•   Usage: Butterbur supplements or extracts.

•   Patients should follow both the recommended dosage written on the product label while healthcare providers can also provide professional advice for dosage recommendations.

2. **Quercetin**

•   The natural antihistamine properties of quercetin help decrease allergic reactions.

•   Quercetin supplements and onions alongside apples and berries function as valid usage for quercetin anti-allergic benefits.

•   You should use the levels of medication indicated on the package label while also seeking guidance from a healthcare provider.

3. **Stinging Nettle**

•   Chioccchio extract provides allergic patients relief through symptom reduction of hay fever along with allergies.

•   People can use stinging nettle as tea and capsules along with extracts of stinging nettle for their treatment.

•   Dosages should be followed based on the description provided on product labels, or a healthcare professional should be consulted for guidance.

4. **Ginger**

•   The antioxidant along anti-inflammatory effects of quercetin help patients experience reduced allergy symptoms.

•   Two usage examples of ginger include fresh ginger tea and ginger capsules, as well as adding fresh ginger to meals.

•   The recommended dose is to be included in daily food consumption or taken as a supplement.

5. **Eyebright**

•   Eyebright offers two therapeutic benefits that help relieve both allergic conjunctivitis symptoms and hay fever symptoms.

•   Usage: Eyebright tea, capsules, or tincture.

•   The recommended amount of medication corresponds to information found on product labels and healthcare provider recommendations.

Dietary Changes to Alleviate Allergies

Anti-Inflammatory Foods

1. **Fruits and Vegetables**

•   Food sources with vitamins and minerals along with antioxidants provide health benefits and inflammatory response reduction.

- Examples: Berries, leafy greens, bell peppers, carrots, tomatoes.

2. **Healthy Fats**

- Essential fatty acids integrate anti-inflammatory compounds into their structure, specifically with omega-3 fatty acids showing these properties.

- Sources: Avocados, nuts, seeds, olive oil, fatty fish (salmon, mackerel, sardines).

3. **Whole Grains**

- The consumption of whole grains can provide necessary nutrients together with fiber, which maintains body health.

- Sources: Brown rice, quinoa, oats, whole wheat.

4. **Probiotic-Rich Foods**

- Foods that support gut health provide vital anti-inflammatory properties that reduce allergy symptoms while reducing inflammation in the body.

- Sources: Yogurt, kefir, sauerkraut, kimchi, miso.

5. **Herbs and Spices**

- Procured from turmeric, ginger, garlic, and cinnamon plants, such foods possess anti-inflammatory compounds that promote body wellness.

- Examples: Turmeric, ginger, garlic, cinnamon.

Foods to Avoid

1. **Processed Foods**

- The food contains fat-filled unwanted substances such as sugar and additives that cause inflammation.

- Processed edibles such as fast food, packaged snacks, and sugary cereals represent examples of these types of food choices.

2. **Dairy Products**

- The consumption of certain foods leads to worse allergy symptoms by intensifying mucus production in specific individuals.

- Alternatives: Plant-based milk, lactose-free dairy products.

3. **Sugary Foods and Beverages**

- Consuming too much sugar causes individuals to gain weight as it triggers inflammatory reactions in the body.

- Examples: Sodas, candies, and pastries.

Lifestyle Changes for Allergy Management

Regular Physical Activity

- The practice of physical exercise brings multiple advantages, including better physical health with decreased stress levels that additionally reduce allergy symptoms.

- The combination of walking, jogging, swimming, cycling, and yoga, along with running and skating, provides suitable exercises.

- People should exercise for 30 minutes at a moderate intensity, approximately five to six days throughout the week.

Stress Management

- The practice reduces stress effects on total health while strengthening immunity.

- Strengthen your relaxation methods through meditation and deep breathing exercises in combination with yoga and mindfulness practice.

- Makers of stress management techniques should integrate them as everyday habits into their daily schedule.

Adequate Sleep

- The goal should be to maintain regular quality sleep because it supports total health outcomes together with allergy symptom relief.

- Creating a fixed sleep pattern along with comfortable sleeping conditions represents part of the routine that should include calming activities before bedtime.

- Your objective should be seven to nine hours each night of excellent sleep duration.

Hydration

- Gaining enough hydration benefits your general health, simultaneously decreasing the symptoms of allergies.

- The daily water intake should consist of many bottled drinks and eating fruits and vegetables that hydrate your body.

- Additional Supportive Practices

Air Purifiers

- Using air purifiers allows users to remove allergens together with dust and air pollution from their home environment.

- Air purifiers with HEPA filters should be used for better indoor air quality.

Regular Cleaning

- The presence of these products minimizes the buildup of dust along with mold and different allergies.

- To minimize allergens, you should vacuum all surfaces using HEPA filtration while performing regular dusting and frequent washing of all bedding.

Ventilation

- The installation of strategic ventilation systems enables better flow of air and decreases indoor air pollutants alongside it.

- Your home requires open windows with exhaust fan usage and sufficient ventilation, as recommended.

Natural Cleaning Products

- Natural cleaning products yield the advantage of minimizing harmful chemical and irritant contact.

- Recommendations: Use natural or non-toxic cleaning products.

Conclusion

Effective allergy management requires patients to determine their allergens while eliminating them from their environment using herbal treatments and eating different foods while practicing healthy habits. Your overall well-being, alongside allergy symptom alleviation, becomes possible through consuming anti-inflammatory foods while integrating herbal therapies and maintaining proper physical activity and stress control, together with clean and ventilated living conditions. A comprehensive strategy based on natural solutions supports both long-term health and effective allergy symptom relief.

27. Energizing Breakfast Recipes

Health and daily energy levels depend on consuming an energizing nutritional breakfast in the morning. A recommendation to begin the day with whole, unprocessed foods supports a nutritious and balanced diet. The guide presents simple yet satisfying breakfast ideas that increase energy while maintaining your hunger control until lunchtime.

1. Berry and Spinach Smoothie Bowl

Ingredients:

- 1 cup fresh spinach
- 1 banana
- 1 cup mixed berries (blueberries, strawberries, raspberries)
- 1 cup almond milk (or any plant-based milk)
- 1 tablespoon chia seeds
- 1 tablespoon almond butter
- Toppings: sliced banana, fresh berries, granola, shredded coconut

Instructions:

1. Blend spinach together with a banana, mixed berries, and almond milk, followed by almond butter and chia seeds. Blend until smooth.

2. Use a bowl to pour your smoothie, then decorate it with sliced banana together with fresh berries, granola, and shredded coconut.

3. Enjoy immediately.

Benefits:

- Rich in antioxidants, vitamins, and minerals.

- This drink combination gives you essential fiber alongside healthy fats and proteins, which help maintain your energy level.

2. Avocado Toast with Eggs

Ingredients:

- 1 ripe avocado
- 2 slices of whole-grain bread
- 2 eggs
- Salt and pepper to taste
- Optional toppings: cherry tomatoes, radishes, microgreens, hot sauce

Instructions:

1. Toast the whole grain bread until golden brown.

2. As the bread toasts, simply mix avocado with salt and pepper for seasoning.

3. Cook your eggs according to your taste until they reach the desired consistency.

4. Place the mashed avocado over your toasted bread before using it.

5. Position the cooked eggs and optional toppings on top of the bread.

6. Serve immediately.

Benefits:

- High in healthy fats, fiber, and protein.
- This food offers persistent power combined with extended feelings of satiation.

3. Overnight Chia Pudding

Ingredients:

- 1/4 cup chia seeds
- 1 cup almond milk (or any plant-based milk)
- 1 tablespoon maple syrup or honey
- 1/2 teaspoon vanilla extract
- Toppings: fresh berries, sliced banana, nuts, seeds

Instructions:

1. Place the chia seeds together with the almond milk along with maple syrup and vanilla extract into a bowl or jar, then stir well. Stir well.

2. Place the mixture in the refrigerator overnight while it needs at least 4 hours for storage.

3. Stir your chia pudding before daybreak then include extra liquid if you need to achieve your preferred consistency.

4. Place the dish with fresh berries alongside sliced bananas and additional nuts and seeds on top.

5. Enjoy immediately.

Benefits:

- Rich in omega-3 fatty acids, fiber, and protein.
- The preparation of this breakfast can occur in advance so you have a ready-to-eat nutritious meal for the day.

4. Greek Yogurt Parfait

Ingredients:

- 1 cup Greek yogurt
- 1/2 cup granola

- 1 cup mixed fresh berries
- 1 tablespoon honey or maple syrup
- Optional toppings: nuts, seeds, shredded coconut

Instructions:

1. In a glass or bowl, layer the Greek yogurt, granola, and mixed berries.
2. Drizzle with honey or maple syrup.
3. Add any optional toppings.
4. Serve immediately.

Benefits:

- High in protein, probiotics, and antioxidants.
- The meal offers quick preparation followed by a prolonged energy supply.

5. Quinoa Breakfast Bowl

Ingredients:

- 1/2 cup cooked quinoa
- 1/2 cup almond milk (or any plant-based milk)
- 1 tablespoon almond butter
- 1 tablespoon chia seeds
- 1 tablespoon honey or maple syrup
- 1/2 teaspoon cinnamon
- Toppings: sliced banana, fresh berries, nuts, seeds

Instructions:

1. Add the hot cooked quinoa to a small pot containing almond milk while heating on medium heat. Heat the mixture at medium temperature until it reaches a warm state.

2. Blend the mixture of almond butter with chia seeds, followed by honey or maple syrup and cinnamon into the pot.

3. Place sliced banana and fresh berries alongside nuts and seeds as topping over the mixture in a separate bowl.

4. Serve immediately.

Benefits:

- Rich in protein, fiber, and essential nutrients.

- This menu option provides consistent energy while maintaining your hunger control throughout the day.

6. Oatmeal with Nuts and Berries

Ingredients:

- 1 cup rolled oats
- 2 cups water or almond milk
- 1 tablespoon chia seeds
- 1/2 teaspoon cinnamon
- 1 tablespoon honey or maple syrup
- Toppings: fresh berries, sliced banana, nuts, seeds

Instructions:

1. Combine water or almond milk in a pot for boiling preparation.

2. Pour the ingredients of rolled oats and chia seeds with cinnamon into the pot. Decrease the heat to low temperature and let the mixture cook while occasionally stirring for 5-7 minutes.

3. After heating, remove the pot from the stove and mix the honey or maple syrup into the mixture.

4. Place the mixture in a bowl and decorate it with fresh berries together with sliced bananas, nuts, and seeds.

5. Serve immediately.

Benefits:

- High in fiber, protein, and antioxidants.

- This dish offers a continuous source of energy together with digestive system wellness benefits.

7. Veggie-Packed Omelette

Ingredients:

- 3 eggs
- 1/4 cup diced bell peppers
- 1/4 cup diced onions
- 1/4 cup spinach
- 1/4 cup diced tomatoes
- 1 tablespoon olive oil
- Salt and pepper to taste
- Optional toppings: avocado, salsa, cheese

Instructions:

1. Combine eggs and salt with pepper in a bowl while stirring until smooth.

2. Place olive oil in a non-stick skillet, then heat it on medium heat.

3. Add all diced bell peppers alongside onions, spinach, and tomatoes to the medium-heat skillet. Cook the vegetables until they reach tenderness during sautéing.

4. Correctly pour the eggs onto the vegetable mixture then let the eggs become set throughout cooking.

5. Move the omelet half into the middle and then shift it to the plate.

6. Put optional topping ingredients onto your dish, then serve without delay.

Benefits:

• These pastries conceal a nutritious protein source along with numerous vital nutrients and valuable minerals obtained from vegetables.

• The dish delivers continuous energy power while supporting your muscle strength.

Conclusion

Your day begins with success once you start it by eating an energizing breakfast that supports your energy needs along with your health system. Wellness and daytime energy rely on consuming unprocessed natural foods, balanced with protein, healthy fats, and carbohydrates as part of a holistic approach to health.

28. Revitalizing Lunch Recipes

Your day requires an energizing lunch to maintain stability in your energy supply while delivering valuable nutrients for your health. Whole, unprocessed foods should serve as the foundation of daily lunchtime meals to support overall health and well-being. Practical meal recipes here are presented with nutritional benefits that restore both energy and bodily health.

1. Quinoa and Veggie Salad

Ingredients:

- 1 cup cooked quinoa
- 1 cup mixed greens (spinach, arugula, kale)
- 1/2 cup cherry tomatoes, halved
- 1/2 cup cucumber, diced
- 1/4 cup red bell pepper, diced
- 1/4 cup red onion, thinly sliced
- 1/4 cup feta cheese (optional)
- 2 tablespoons olive oil
- 1 tablespoon lemon juice
- 1 teaspoon Dijon mustard
- Salt and pepper to taste

Instructions:

1. A large mixing bowl contains cooked quinoa joined with mixed greens and cherry tomatoes combined with cucumber, red bell pepper, and red onion.

2. Whisk an olive oil mixture that includes lemon juice and Dijon mustard, as well as a seasoning of salt and pepper, in a small mixing bowl.

3. Combine all contents by adding dressing to the salad, then toss until everything is well mixed.

4. Add crumbled feta cheese only when serving.

5. Serve immediately.

Benefits:

- High in protein, fiber, and essential nutrients.
- The combination supplies continuous energy while maintaining body wellness.

2. Mediterranean Chickpea Salad

Ingredients:

- 1 can (15 oz) chickpeas, drained and rinsed
- 1/2 cup cherry tomatoes, halved
- 1/2 cup cucumber, diced
- 1/4 cup red onion, thinly sliced
- 1/4 cup Kalamata olives, pitted and halved
- 1/4 cup feta cheese (optional)
- 2 tablespoons olive oil
- 1 tablespoon red wine vinegar
- 1 teaspoon dried oregano
- Salt and pepper to taste

Instructions:

1. A large bowl contains the mixture of chickpeas with cherry tomatoes alongside cucumber and, red onion and Kalamata olives.

2. Stir the mixture of olive oil with red wine vinegar along with oregano and salt and pepper in a separate bowl.

3. Mix the salad by adding dressing from step 2 throughout step 1.

4. Place the feta cheese on top if using it as an addition.

5. The dish should be consumed immediately but can also remain refrigerated until serving time.

Benefits:

- Rich in fiber, protein, and healthy fats.
- The nutritional compound contains benefits for heart health and sustains energy levels without interruption.

3. Sweet Potato and Black Bean Tacos

Ingredients:

- 2 medium sweet potatoes, peeled and diced
- 1 can (15 oz) black beans, drained and rinsed
- 1 tablespoon olive oil
- 1 teaspoon ground cumin
- 1 teaspoon smoked paprika
- 1/2 teaspoon chili powder
- Salt and pepper to taste
- 8 small corn tortillas
- Toppings: avocado, salsa, chopped cilantro, lime wedges

Instructions:

1. Preheat the oven to 400°F (200°C).

2. Combine the sweet potatoes with oil and season them with cumin, paprika, chili powder, and salt and pepper together.

3. Place sweet potato portions onto a baking sheet then let them roast between 20 and 25 minutes until they become tender and lightly crispy.

4. Heat black beans at medium temperature until they become warm in a small cooking pot.

5. Heat the corn tortillas through dry pan cooking or the microwave method.

6. Place the divided sweet potatoes and black beans equally in the tortillas to assemble each taco.

7. Place avocado next to the salsa and lime juice on top, followed by chopped cilantro.

8. Serve immediately.

Benefits:

- High in fiber, vitamins, and minerals.
- Black beans supply steady energy while they help maintain digestive wellness.

4. Lentil and Vegetable Soup

Ingredients:

- 1 cup dried lentils, rinsed
- 1 tablespoon olive oil
- 1 onion, diced
- 2 carrots, diced
- 2 celery stalks, diced
- 3 cloves garlic, minced
- 1 can (14.5 oz) diced tomatoes
- 6 cups vegetable broth

- 1 teaspoon dried thyme
- 1 teaspoon dried basil
- 2 cups spinach, roughly chopped
- Salt and pepper to taste

Instructions:

1. Heat olive oil in a large pot at medium temperature.

2. The pot receives onion and carrot, then celery pieces. The vegetable combination requires sautéing until they achieve tenderness for 5-7 minutes.

3. The garlic goes into the pot for one more minute of cooking.

4. Put the diced tomatoes together with vegetable broth into the pot, followed by lentils and additions of dried thyme and dried basil.

5. The mixture needs to reach boiling point before adjusting the heat to low and letting it cook for 25-30 minutes until the lentils soften.

6. Young spinach leaves need 2-3 minutes to wilt while they cook with the other ingredients.

7. There should be a final addition of salt and pepper for flavor adjustment.

8. Serve hot.

Benefits:

- High in protein, fiber, and essential nutrients.
- The meal offers sustained energy support to strengthen immune function.

5. Hummus and Veggie Wrap

Ingredients:

- 1 large whole-grain tortilla

- 1/2 cup hummus
- 1/4 cup shredded carrots
- 1/4 cup sliced cucumber
- 1/4 cup sliced bell peppers
- 1/4 cup baby spinach
- 1/4 cup alfalfa sprouts
- 1 tablespoon sunflower seeds
- Salt and pepper to taste

Instructions:

1. Apply a thin and uniform layer of hummus on top of the tortilla.

2. Place shredded carrots, followed by sliced cucumber, then bell peppers and baby spinach, before adding alfalfa sprouts on the hummus.

3. Season the mixture with pepper and salt and sprinkle with sunflower seeds afterward.

4. After folding the tortilla tightly, cut it into two parts.

5. The dish is ready to serve immediately, or you can use foil to make it portable for lunch outside.

Benefits:

- Rich in fiber, healthy fats, and essential nutrients.
- The combination offers long-lasting energy as well as promotes digestive health.

6. Greek Quinoa Bowl

Ingredients:

- 1 cup cooked quinoa
- 1/2 cup cherry tomatoes, halved

- 1/2 cup cucumber, diced
- 1/4 cup Kalamata olives, pitted and halved
- 1/4 cup red onion, thinly sliced
- 1/4 cup feta cheese (optional)
- 2 tablespoons olive oil
- 1 tablespoon lemon juice
- 1 teaspoon dried oregano
- Salt and pepper to taste

Instructions:

1. Mix all ingredients, starting with cooked quinoa followed by cherry tomatoes then continue with cucumber and Kalamata olives and finishing with red onion in a large mixing bowl.

2. Mix all ingredients in a small bowl where you combine 2 tablespoons of olive oil with the lemon juice along with dried oregano, salt and black pepper.

3. Add the dressing to the quinoa mix, then mix all ingredients until they are evenly coated.

4. Finish the salad with feta cheese as an optional topping.

5. Serve this dish immediately because it remains fresh up to a point where proper refrigeration extends its eating time.

Benefits:

- High in protein, fiber, and healthy fats.
- The grain delivers both health benefits and prolonged energy maintenance.

7. Avocado and Chickpea Salad Sandwich

Ingredients:

- 1 ripe avocado
- 1 can (15 oz) chickpeas, drained and rinsed
- 1 tablespoon lemon juice
- 1/4 cup red onion, finely chopped
- 1/4 cup celery, finely chopped
- 1/4 cup cilantro, chopped
- Salt and pepper to taste
- Whole grain bread

Instructions:

1. Mix the avocado and chickpeas in a medium-sized bowl until both ingredients become smooth together.

2. Mix all components together in the medium bowl of the mixture including celery along with red onion, lemon juice, and cilantro.

3. Adjust the dishes with salt followed by black pepper according to personal choice before consumption.

4. Place the chickpea avocado mixture across whole grain bread pieces.

5. Serve immediately.

Benefits:

- High in healthy fats, fiber, and protein.
- This combination delivers sustainable energy, and it helps support digestive functions.

Conclusion

Your energy stability and nutritional needs for good health will receive support from a rejuvenating lunch period. Early-stage health depends on consuming unprocessed whole foods that blend protein with healthy fats and carbs while promoting daily vitality.

29. Nourishing Dinner Recipes

Your healthy day concludes with a well-balanced dinner that gives your body the needed nutrients for healing as well as recovery processes. Evening meals should consist of complete, unprocessed whole foods to support optimal digestion and overall well-being. A practical set of delicious evening recipes exists in this guide, which promotes health and nourishment.

1. Baked Salmon with Quinoa and Steamed Vegetables

Ingredients:

- 2 salmon fillets
- 1 cup quinoa
- 2 cups broccoli florets
- 2 cups carrots, sliced
- 2 tablespoons olive oil
- 1 lemon, sliced
- 1 teaspoon dried dill
- Salt and pepper to taste

Instructions:

1. Preheat the oven to 400°F (200°C).

2. Salmon fillets should be placed on a baking sheet that contains parchment paper. Dress the salmon with olive oil before adding salt, white pepper, dried dill mixtures and artfully placing lemon slices on top.

3. The salmon will need about 15 to 20 minutes of baking time until it turns fully cooked while remaining flaky.

4. The salmon should be placed in the oven when you begin preparing the quinoa according to package guidelines.

5. Boil the broccoli and carrots using steam until they reach the desired tenderness for 5-7 minutes.

6. The dish consists of baked salmon presented above quinoa together with steamed vegetables.

Benefits:

- High in protein, omega-3 fatty acids, and essential nutrients.

- Heart health benefits, together with long-lasting energy support, are among its advantages.

2. Chickpea and Spinach Curry

Ingredients:

- 1 can (15 oz) chickpeas, drained and rinsed

- 2 cups fresh spinach, roughly chopped

- 1 onion, diced

- 2 cloves garlic, minced

- 1 tablespoon ginger, minced

- 1 can (14.5 oz) diced tomatoes

- 1 can (14 oz) coconut milk

- 1 tablespoon curry powder

- 1 teaspoon ground cumin

- 1 teaspoon ground coriander

- 1 tablespoon olive oil

- Salt and pepper to taste

- Fresh cilantro, chopped (for garnish)

- Cooked brown rice (for serving)

Instructions:

1. Heat olive oil in a large pot at medium temperature.

2. Put the diced onion in the pot to cook for 5 minutes until it becomes translucent.

3. Allow the garlic-ginger mixture to remain in the heat for 1 minute before continuing.

4. Combine the pot contents with curry powder and, ground cumin and ground coriander before cooking the spices for 1-2 minutes until their smell becomes stronger.

5. Stir in the precooked diced tomatoes together with coconut milk and chickpeas. The mixture synergizes its flavors during a 10-15 minute simmer period.

6. After adding the chopped spinach to the pot continue cooking until the leaves become tender through 2-3 minutes.

7. Testing the dish for salt and pepper adds the perfect flavor.

8. Set the curry meal over brown rice with fresh cilantro leaves as garnish.

Benefits:

- Rich in protein, fiber, and anti-inflammatory compounds.
- The dish promotes digestive well-being while delivering gradual energy release.

3. Stuffed Bell Peppers

Ingredients:

- 4 large bell peppers, tops cut off and seeds removed
- 1 cup cooked quinoa

- 1 can (15 oz) black beans, drained and rinsed
- 1 cup corn kernels
- 1 cup diced tomatoes
- 1 onion, diced
- 2 cloves garlic, minced
- 1 teaspoon ground cumin
- 1 teaspoon smoked paprika
- 1 tablespoon olive oil
- Salt and pepper to taste
- Fresh cilantro, chopped (for garnish)

Instructions:

1. Preheat the oven to 375°F (190°C).

2. Heat the skillet along with olive oil at a medium temperature level.

3. The diced onions need to saute until translucent while heating at medium heat for 5 minutes.

4. Continue heat until garlic stays in the pot for 1 more minute.

5. Pour the cooked quinoa together with black beans, corn, diced tomatoes, ground cumin, and smoked paprika into the mixture. Heat the mixture to a full temperature during a 5-7 minute cooking period.

6. Test the dish with salt and pepper according to your preference.

7. Put the quinoa mixture inside the bell peppers, then arrange them in a baking dish.

8. Place foil over the dish before baking it for 30 to 35 minutes until the peppers achieve tenderness.

9. Serve the dish while garnishing it with fresh cilantro leaves.

Benefits:

- High in protein, fiber, and essential nutrients.
- The mixture delivers steady energy to your body and promotes good digestion.

4. Lemon Garlic Shrimp with Zucchini Noodles

Ingredients:

- 1 lb shrimp, peeled and deveined
- 4 zucchini, spiralized into noodles
- 2 tablespoons olive oil
- 3 cloves garlic, minced
- 1 lemon, juiced and zested
- 1/4 cup fresh parsley, chopped
- Salt and pepper to taste
- Red pepper flakes (optional)

Instructions:

1. A large skillet requires preheating with one tablespoon of olive oil at medium temperature.

2. Sprinkle the shrimp with salt while adding pepper and red pepper flakes until the desired taste is reached. Cook the shrimp for 2 to 3 minutes while allowing each side to turn pink and opacity to appear. Set the shrimp next to the skillet for the moment.

3. Place the other tablespoon of olive oil into the same skillet, followed by freshly minced garlic. Sauté until fragrant, about 1 minute.

4. Transfer the zucchini noodles into the skillet and allow them to become barely tender during a 2–3-minute cooking time.

5. Stir the shrimp together with lemon juice and chopped parsley while also adding lemon zest to the skillet. Toss to combine.

6. Serve immediately.

Benefits:

- The dish contains minimal carbohydrates but abundant nutrients together with protein.

- Eating this meal provides heart health benefits along with energy and remains mild on the body.

5. Vegan Lentil Bolognese

Ingredients:

- 1 cup dried lentils, rinsed
- 1 onion, diced
- 2 carrots, diced
- 2 celery stalks, diced
- 3 cloves garlic, minced
- 1 can (28 oz) crushed tomatoes
- 2 tablespoons tomato paste
- 1 teaspoon dried basil
- 1 teaspoon dried oregano
- 1 tablespoon olive oil
- Salt and pepper to taste
- Fresh basil, chopped (for garnish)
- Cooked whole-grain pasta or zucchini noodles (for serving)

Instructions:

1. Heat a large pot with olive oil at medium temperature.

2. The diced onion, celery, and carrot pieces should be added to the pot. Cook the vegetables by sautéing them until they become tender for 5 to 7 minutes.

3. Cook the garlic for one minute after adding it to the mixture.

4. Combine all the ingredients of lentils with crushed tomatoes and tomato paste and add dried basil and dried oregano. Place the mixture on heat until boiling before lowering the heat intensity to cook the lentils until they become tender for 25-30 minutes.

5. Taste the dish with salt and pepper according to your preference.

6. The lentil bolognese should be served with either whole-grain pasta or zucchini noodles.

7. Serve the dish while topping it with fresh basil.

Benefits:

- High in protein, fiber, and essential nutrients.
- The combination delivers nutrients that promote digestive wellness alongside long-lasting energy benefits.

6. Grilled Chicken with Avocado Salsa

Ingredients:

- 2 boneless, skinless chicken breasts
- 2 tablespoons olive oil
- 1 teaspoon ground cumin
- 1 teaspoon smoked paprika
- Salt and pepper to taste
- 2 avocados, diced

- 1/2 red onion, diced
- 1 cup cherry tomatoes, halved
- 1/4 cup fresh cilantro, chopped
- 1 lime, juiced

Instructions:

1. Preheat the grill to medium-high heat.

2. A small mixing bowl contains olive oil along with ground cumin, smoked paprika, salt, and pepper combined into it. You should apply this mixture to each chicken breast.

3. The chicken needs to grill for 6-8 minutes before it reaches doneness when both sides are cooked and the juices become clear.

4. Use your grill time to mix diced avocados with red onion and cherry tomatoes, along with cilantro and lime juice, in a bowl to prepare the avocado salsa. Taste the chicken with salt and pepper for the desired seasoning level.

5. Present the grilled chicken breasts accompanied with avocado salsa.

Benefits:

- High in protein, healthy fats, and essential nutrients.
- The product promotes muscle health while delivering continuous fuel endurance.

7. Sweet Potato and Black Bean Enchiladas

Ingredients:

- 2 large sweet potatoes, peeled and diced
- 1 can (15 oz) black beans, drained and rinsed
- 1 onion, diced

- 2 cloves garlic, minced
- 1 cup corn kernels
- 1 can (15 oz) enchilada sauce
- 8 whole grain tortillas
- 1 cup shredded cheese (optional)
- 2 tablespoons olive oil
- Salt and pepper to taste
- Fresh cilantro, chopped (for garnish)

Instructions:

1. Preheat the oven to 375°F (190°C).

2. Heat medium heat on a large skillet until the olive oil becomes ready. Heat the skillet with olive oil, then cook the diced onion until it becomes transparent after five minutes.

3. Cook the garlic for a further minute until it reaches the desired consistency.

4. The diced sweet potatoes require 10-12 minutes of cooking time until they become tender during this process in the skillet.

5. After heating the mixture with the black beans and corn, it should reach the desired temperature. Dress the mixture with salt and pepper as per your preference.

6. Set up a baking dish by using an even coating of enchilada sauce at the bottom.

7. Place the delicious sweet potato filling into the tortillas, then fold them into rolls. Arrange the complete tortillas with the joined edge facing downwards in the baking dish.

8. Distribute the leftover enchilada sauce across the surface before finishing it with shredded cheese if you choose to use it.

9. Place the pan under foil as you bake it for 20-25 minutes until both contents heat fully and the cheese becomes melted.

10. Serve the dish when garnished with fresh cilantro leaves.

30. Healthy Snacks and Sides

Food that supports energy levels and overall wellness should be part of your diet in order to avoid excessive eating during main meals. Snacks and side dishes should include complete, unprocessed foods.

This guide brings readers simple recipes of nutritious snacks and accompanying dishes to provide sustained nourishment.

Healthy Snacks

1. Hummus and Veggie Sticks

Ingredients:

- 1 can (15 oz) chickpeas, drained and rinsed
- 1/4 cup tahini
- 2 tablespoons olive oil
- 2 tablespoons lemon juice
- 2 cloves garlic, minced
- 1/2 teaspoon ground cumin
- Salt and pepper to taste
- Water, as needed for consistency
- Veggie sticks: carrots, celery, cucumber, bell peppers

Instructions:

1. Put the chickpeas together with tahini along with olive oil and lemon juice into the food processor while adding garlic mixed with ground cumin and salt and pepper to taste.

2. The food processor needs continuous operation to achieve smooth results while you gradually add water to attain the ideal texture.

3. An assorted array of veggie sticks should accompany the hummus when serving.

Benefits:

• High in fiber, healthy fats, and protein.

• The mixture supports digestion while delivering a steady power supply to the body.

2. Greek Yogurt and Berry Parfait

Ingredients:

• 1 cup Greek yogurt

• 1/2 cup mixed fresh berries (blueberries, strawberries, raspberries)

• 1/4 cup granola

• 1 tablespoon honey or maple syrup (optional)

• 1 tablespoon chia seeds

Instructions:

1. Prepare the parfait by arranging Greek yogurt followed by mixed berries and granola on top with chia seeds in a glass or bowl.

2. Culminate your dessert by drizzling either honey or maple syrup.

3. Serve immediately.

Benefits:

• High in protein, antioxidants, and fiber.

• The combination of components helps improve digestive health and gives the body ongoing sources of energy.

3. Almond Butter and Apple Slices

Ingredients:

- 1 apple, sliced
- 2 tablespoons almond butter
- 1 tablespoon chia seeds or flaxseeds (optional)
- 1/4 teaspoon ground cinnamon (optional)

Instructions:

1. Set the apple pieces on a serving plate before continuing.
2. Spread almond butter on each slice.
3. Chia seeds, together with flaxseeds and cinnamon ground powder, can enhance the dish if added as toppings.
4. Serve immediately.

Benefits:

- High in healthy fats, fiber, and protein.
- The combination supports both overall health and delivers the body steady power for energy activity.

4. Trail Mix

Ingredients:

- 1/2 cup almonds
- 1/2 cup walnuts
- 1/2 cup cashews
- 1/2 cup pumpkin seeds
- 1/2 cup dried cranberries or raisins
- 1/4 cup dark chocolate chips (optional)

Instructions:

1. Mix all ingredients, including almonds, walnuts, cashews, pumpkin seeds, dried cranberries, or raisins, alongside dark chocolate chips in a large bowl.

2. Place the ingredients into a mixture bowl, then store them in a closed container.

3. Enjoy as a healthy snack.

Benefits:

- Rich in healthy fats, protein, and antioxidants.

These foods supply continuous energy while benefiting heart wellness.

5. Avocado Toast

Ingredients:

- 1 ripe avocado
- 2 slices whole grain bread
- 1/2 lemon, juiced
- Salt and pepper to taste
- Optional toppings: cherry tomatoes, radishes, microgreens, red pepper flakes

Instructions:

1. Toast the whole grain bread until golden brown.

2. The avocado should be mashed while the bread toasts, then combined with lemon juice and seasoning.

3. Smooth avocado puree should be spread over the toasted bread.

4. Add optional toppings as desired.

5. Serve immediately.

Benefits:

- High in healthy fats, fiber, and essential nutrients.
- The combination benefits both heart wellness and offers an extended energy supply.

Healthy Sides

1. Roasted Brussels Sprouts

Ingredients:

- 1 lb Brussels sprouts, trimmed and halved
- 2 tablespoons olive oil
- Salt and pepper to taste
- 1/2 teaspoon garlic powder (optional)
- 1/2 teaspoon smoked paprika (optional)

Instructions:

1. Preheat the oven to 400°F (200°C).
2. Marinate Brussels sprouts with olive oil and season them using salt pepper along with garlic powder and smoked paprika.
3. Put the Brussels sprouts onto a baking tray while keeping them in a single layer.
4. Let the Brussels sprouts roast for 20-25 minutes in the oven until they become tender while developing crispy sections around their edges.
5. Serve immediately.

Benefits:

- High in fiber, vitamins, and antioxidants.
- Brussels sprouts offer benefits for digestive health as well as general wellness.

2. Quinoa Salad

Ingredients:

- 1 cup cooked quinoa
- 1/2 cup cherry tomatoes, halved
- 1/2 cup cucumber, diced
- 1/4 cup red onion, finely chopped
- 1/4 cup feta cheese (optional)
- 2 tablespoons olive oil
- 1 tablespoon lemon juice
- 1 teaspoon dried oregano
- Salt and pepper to taste

Instructions:

1. The mixture begins with a bowl that holds the cooked quinoa together with all the ingredients, including cherry tomatoes, cucumber, red onion, and feta cheese.

2. Mix all ingredients of olive oil and lemon juice, dried oregano, salt, and pepper in a small bowl.

3. Combine all ingredients in the quinoa salad bowl and dress it with the prepared dressing immediately.

4. The dish requires immediate serving, but you can store it in refrigeration before you eat.

Benefits:

- High in protein, fiber, and essential nutrients.
- The combination helps build health while supplying long-lasting energy to the body.

3. Steamed Asparagus with Lemon

Ingredients:

- 1 bunch asparagus, trimmed
- 1 tablespoon olive oil
- 1 lemon, juiced and zested
- Salt and pepper to taste

Instructions:

1. Cook the asparagus in steam heat until it reaches a tender consistency for 5 to 7 minutes.

2. Luxuriate the steamed asparagus directly onto a decorative serving dish.

3. Drizzle with olive oil, lemon juice, and lemon zest.

4. Season with salt and pepper.

5. Serve immediately.

Benefits:

- High in vitamins, minerals, and antioxidants.
- The dish gives both health benefits and acts as a light, refreshing side plate.

4. Sweet Potato Fries

Ingredients:

- 2 large sweet potatoes, peeled and cut into fries
- 2 tablespoons olive oil
- 1/2 teaspoon paprika
- 1/2 teaspoon garlic powder

- Salt and pepper to taste

Instructions:

1. Preheat the oven to 425°F (220°C).

2. Mix sweet potato fries together with olive oil, followed by seasonings of paprika along with garlic powder and salt and pepper.

3. Set all fried potatoes flat on a baking sheet.

4. Place the sweet potato fries on the baking sheet and bake for 20-25 minutes while you need to flip them at the halfway point until they achieve a crispy golden-brown finish.

5. Serve immediately.

Benefits:

- High in fiber, vitamins, and minerals.
- The food item supplies continuous energy and benefits the stomach system.

5. Greek Salad

Ingredients:

- 1 cucumber, diced
- 1 cup cherry tomatoes, halved
- 1/4 cup red onion, thinly sliced
- 1/4 cup Kalamata olives, pitted and halved
- 1/4 cup feta cheese (optional)
- 2 tablespoons olive oil
- 1 tablespoon red wine vinegar
- 1 teaspoon dried oregano
- Salt and pepper to taste

Instructions:

1. A large mixing bowl contains cucumber chunks together with cherry tomatoes mixed with red onion and Kalamata olives, as well as crumbled feta cheese.

2. A small mixing bowl contains a mixture of olive oil with red wine vinegar, dried oregano, and salt and pepper.

3. Stir the salad until all the ingredients are properly mixed together.

4. Serve immediately.

Benefits:

- High in antioxidants, healthy fats, and essential nutrients.
- The mixture supports heart health and offers a pleasant, refreshing side dish.

Conclusion

Adding nutritious small meals and sides to your dining routines helps keep your energy steady and enhances your general health. You can find nutritious and flavorful snacks and side dishes by choosing natural, unprocessed foods that bring benefits to your health. This approach combines natural foods with high nutrient values to promote long-term vitality and overall well-being.

31. Wholesome Desserts

Dessert consumption should not interfere with your health improvement objectives. The importance of using only pure, unprocessed ingredients in all sweet items is strongly emphasized. The guide presents delectable yet nourishing sweet recipes that also supply vital nutrients to maintain your health.

1. Dark Chocolate Avocado Mousse

Ingredients:

- 2 ripe avocados
- 1/4 cup unsweetened cocoa powder
- 1/4 cup honey or maple syrup
- 1/4 cup almond milk (or any plant-based milk)
- 1 teaspoon vanilla extract
- A pinch of salt

Instructions:

1. The food processor allows you to mix avocados with cocoa powder along with honey or maple syrup, almond milk, vanilla extract, and salt.

2. Process until smooth and creamy.

3. The divided mousse should rest in refrigeration for a minimum of 30 minutes before you serve it.

4. Optional: Garnish with fresh berries or a sprinkle of cocoa nibs.

Benefits:

- Rich in healthy fats, antioxidants, and fiber.

- The mixture delivers rich creaminess through natural ingredients that omit both dairy content and sugar additives.

2. Berry Chia Pudding

Ingredients:

- 1/4 cup chia seeds
- 1 cup almond milk (or any plant-based milk)
- 1 tablespoon honey or maple syrup
- 1 teaspoon vanilla extract
- 1 cup mixed fresh berries (blueberries, strawberries, raspberries)

Instructions:

1. Stir the mixture of chia seeds along with almond milk and either honey or maple syrup and vanilla extract in a bowl or jar before placing it in the refrigerator. Stir well.

2. Placing the mixture in the refrigerator allows it to develop its flavors for a minimum of 4 hours, but leaving it overnight will optimize its taste.

3. Mix the chia pudding at the start of the day, then add extra liquid if you want a thinner texture.

4. Top with mixed fresh berries.

5. Serve immediately.

Benefits:

- High in omega-3 fatty acids, fiber, and antioxidants.
- This recipe offers a simple preparation method with an advanced preparation option for quick, nutritious dessert service.

3. Baked Apples with Cinnamon and Walnuts

Ingredients:

- 4 medium apples
- 1/4 cup walnuts, chopped
- 1/4 cup raisins
- 1 tablespoon honey or maple syrup
- 1 teaspoon ground cinnamon
- 1/2 teaspoon ground nutmeg
- 1/2 cup water

Instructions:

1. Preheat the oven to 350°F (175°C).

2. Cut a hole through each apple while keeping its bottom intact as a support for filling.

3. A small bowl contains a mixture made with walnuts and raisins, along with honey or maple syrup together with cinnamon and nutmeg.

4. Add the mixture to the hollow-cored apples.

5. Add the apples to a baking dish followed by adding water to the base of it.

6. Place the dish in the oven at 350 degrees Fahrenheit for thirty to thirty-five minutes until the apples become soft.

7. Serve this dish hot with an optional addition of Greek yogurt on the side.

Benefits:

- Rich in fiber, vitamins, and healthy fats.

- This sweet dessert offers comforting warmth without any refined sugar content.

4. Coconut Bliss Balls

Ingredients:

- 1 cup pitted dates
- 1 cup shredded unsweetened coconut
- 1/2 cup almonds or cashews
- 2 tablespoons cocoa powder
- 1 tablespoon coconut oil
- 1 teaspoon vanilla extract
- A pinch of salt

Instructions:

1. Process all the ingredients, such as dates, along with shredded coconut and almonds or cashews, cocoa powder, coconut oil, vanilla extract, and salt in a food processor until the mixture sticks together.

2. Proceed with blending until the mixture develops into a pasty sticky mass.

3. Shape the mixture into small balls which you should put onto a baking sheet that has parchment paper on it.

4. Let the mixture refrigerate for at least 30 minutes until it reaches serving temperature.

5. Keep the mixture stored in an airtight container in the refrigerator.

Benefits:

- High in fiber, healthy fats, and natural sweetness.

- These snacks supply satisfying energy while delivering a natural boost without including refined sugar.

5. Banana Ice Cream

Ingredients:

- 4 ripe bananas, sliced and frozen
- 1/2 teaspoon vanilla extract
- Optional toppings: chopped nuts, dark chocolate chips, fresh berries

Instructions:

1. A food processor should blend the frozen bananas to generate a smooth puree.

2. Condense the mixture by adding the vanilla extract and blend once more.

3. The frozen dessert is ready as soft serve now, but freezers will produce a firmer texture if left to rest for another hour in a proper container.

4. Options to decorate the frozen treat include nuts, melted dark chocolate, or fresh fruit.

Benefits:

- The mixture offers a sweet, creamy taste while keeping out both added dairy ingredients and sugars.
- Provides a refreshing, guilt-free dessert.

6. Oatmeal Raisin Cookies

Ingredients:

- 1 cup rolled oats
- 1/2 cup almond flour

- 1/2 cup raisins
- 1/4 cup honey or maple syrup
- 1/4 cup coconut oil, melted
- 1 teaspoon vanilla extract
- 1/2 teaspoon ground cinnamon
- 1/4 teaspoon baking soda
- A pinch of salt

Instructions:

1. The first step should be to heat the oven to 350°F (175°C) and place parchment paper on a baking sheet.

2. Place the rolled oats together with almond flour and raisins into a mixing bowl along with cinnamon powder and add baking soda and salt.

3. Both the honey or maple syrup and melted coconut oil mix with the vanilla extract in a separate bowl for use in this recipe.

4. Combine the wet mixture with the dry mixture while stirring until the dough becomes well-mixed.

5. Drop the dough onto the prepared baking sheet using spoonfuls while pressing them slightly flat with a spoon.

6. Place the sheet into the oven for 10-12 minutes until the cookie borders turn golden.

7. Place the baked cookies on the baking tray for several minutes of cooling time before moving them to wire racks for a complete cooling process.

Benefits:

- High in fiber, healthy fats, and natural sweetness.

- The cookies offer a protein-rich tasty delight without including refined sugars or flour.

7. Mango Coconut Chia Pudding

Ingredients:

- 1/4 cup chia seeds
- 1 cup coconut milk
- 1 tablespoon honey or maple syrup
- 1 teaspoon vanilla extract
- 1 ripe mango, diced

Instructions:

1. A bowl or jar containing chia seeds and coconut milk with honey or maple syrup and vanilla extract should be stirred together. Stir well.

2. Put the covered mixture into your refrigerator for a time period of 4 hours minimum or leave it to rest overnight.

3. Mix the chia pudding at dawn while adding additional liquid if required to achieve the preferred texture.

4. Top with diced mango.

5. Serve immediately.

Benefits:

- High in omega-3 fatty acids, fiber, and antioxidants.
- The mixture creates a sweet tropical pudding while offering natural flavor satisfaction.

Conclusion

The combination of healthy ingredients allows you to enjoy enjoyable and beneficial sweet treats. Procuring unprocessed, wholesome components enables you to create sugar-rich dishes that serve your health needs. You can satisfy your desire for sweet treats through these nutritious recipes, which offer multiple tastes and textures. A holistic approach emphasizes that natural, wholesome foods are essential for sustaining long-term health and vitality.

32. Healing Beverages

The consumption of healing beverages supplies basic nutrients while benefiting overall health and supporting natural healing functions in the body. Enhancements in health result from incorporating natural, whole ingredients into beverage preparations.

The guide delivers straightforward recipes that produce nutritious healing drinks that promote your wellness.

1. Turmeric Golden Milk

Ingredients:

- 1 cup almond milk (or any plant-based milk)
- 1 teaspoon ground turmeric
- 1/2 teaspoon ground ginger
- 1/4 teaspoon ground cinnamon
- 1 tablespoon honey or maple syrup (optional)
- A pinch of black pepper
- 1 teaspoon coconut oil (optional)

Instructions:

1. The mixture of almond milk and turmeric, along with ginger, cinnamon, and black pepper, goes into a small saucepan for heating.

2. Heat this mixture on medium heat until it reaches an acceptable temperature that is less than boiling.

3. Stir in honey or maple syrup together with coconut oil after removing the mixture from the heat.

4. Serve the mixture immediately from a mug.

Benefits:

- Anti-inflammatory and antioxidant properties.
- Supports immune health and digestion.

2. Ginger Lemon Tea

Ingredients:

- 1-inch piece of fresh ginger, sliced
- 1 lemon, juiced
- 1 tablespoon honey or maple syrup (optional)
- 2 cups water

Instructions:

1. Put the water into a small pot and let it reach boiling temperature.

2. Pour the sliced ginger into the pot before lowering the heat and allowing it to simmer for 10 minutes. Let it simmer for 10 minutes.

3. Extract the ginger through straining after heat removal from the pot.

4. Mix the liquid with lemon juice along with optional honey or maple syrup.

5. Serve the drink immediately from the mug.

Benefits:

- Anti-inflammatory and antioxidant properties.
- This mixture has two beneficial effects because it supports the digestive process while strengthening your immune system.

3. Green Smoothie

Ingredients:

- 1 cup fresh spinach

- 1 banana
- 1/2 cup frozen mango
- 1/2 cup frozen pineapple
- 1 cup coconut water (or any plant-based milk)
- 1 tablespoon chia seeds (optional)

Instructions:

1. Put the water into a small pot and let it reach boiling temperature.

2. Pour the sliced ginger into the pot before lowering the heat and allowing it to simmer for 10 minutes. Let it simmer for 10 minutes.

3. Extract the ginger through straining after heat removal from the pot.

4. Mix the liquid with lemon juice along with optional honey or maple syrup.

5. Serve the drink immediately from the mug.

Benefits:

- Anti-inflammatory and antioxidant properties.
- This mixture has two beneficial effects because it supports the digestive process while strengthening your immune system.

4. Herbal Immune-Boosting Tea

Ingredients:

- 1 teaspoon dried echinacea
- 1 teaspoon dried elderberries
- 1 teaspoon dried ginger root
- 1 teaspoon dried peppermint leaves
- 2 cups water

- Honey or lemon, to taste (optional)

Instructions:

1. Combine water in a small pot and let it reach boiling temperature.

2. Pour all the echinacea with elderberries into the boiling water and add both ginger root and peppermint leaves.

3. Lower the heat of the mixture and allow the mixture to continue simmering for 10 to 15 minutes.

4. After heating, remove all the herbs through a straining process.

5. Complete the mixture with optional honey or lemon.

6. Pour the mixture into a serving mug while it should be consumed right away.

Benefits:

- Supports immune health and respiratory health.

- The mixture offers both comfort through its relaxing nature and serves as an enjoyable drink.

5. Beetroot and Apple Juice

Ingredients:

- 1 medium beetroot, peeled and chopped
- 2 apples, cored and chopped
- 1-inch piece of fresh ginger
- 1 tablespoon lemon juice
- 1 cup water

Instructions:

1. The blender contains beetroot together with apples and ginger alongside lemon juice and water.

2. Blend until smooth.

3. You should strain the juice once through both a fine mesh strainer and cheesecloth to eliminate pulp.

4. The beverage should be served right after pouring into the glass.

Benefits:

- Rich in antioxidants, vitamins, and minerals.

- Support from this drink benefits liver health and provides increased energy.

6. Matcha Green Tea Latte

Ingredients:

- 1 teaspoon matcha green tea powder

- 1/4 cup hot water (not boiling)

- 3/4 cup almond milk (or any plant-based milk)

- 1 tablespoon honey or maple syrup (optional)

Instructions:

1. Use a small bowl to mix matcha green tea powder with hot water while creating a smooth and frothed texture.

2. Place the almond milk in a small saucepan before heating it to a warm temperature that remains below boiling.

3. Place the matcha mixture into a mug, followed by pouring in the warm almond milk.

4. Finish the mixture by adding honey or maple syrup when desired.

5. Serve immediately.

Benefits:

- Rich in antioxidants and amino acids.

- This beverage delivers light energy increases while helping users remain mentally focused.

7. Detoxifying Cucumber Mint Water

Ingredients:

- 1 cucumber, thinly sliced
- 1/4 cup fresh mint leaves
- 1 lemon, thinly sliced
- 8 cups water

Instructions:

1. A large pitcher contains the ingredients of cucumber slices combined with mint leaves, lemon slices, and water.

2. Set the mixture in the refrigerator for at least one hour to complete the infusion of flavors.

3. Serve the mixture chilled after it is poured into glasses.

Benefits:

- Hydrates and detoxifies the body.
- Refreshing and supporting digestive health.

8. Golden Turmeric Smoothie

Ingredients:

- 1 banana
- 1/2 cup frozen pineapple
- 1/2 teaspoon ground turmeric
- 1/2 teaspoon ground ginger
- 1 cup coconut milk (or any plant-based milk)

- 1 tablespoon chia seeds (optional)
- A pinch of black pepper

Instructions:

1. The blender combines banana and frozen pineapple with turmeric, ginger, coconut milk, chia seeds, along with black pepper.

2. Blend until smooth.

3. Drink the mixture right away through a glass.

Benefits:

- Anti-inflammatory and antioxidant properties.
- The mixture offers sustained energy together with immune health support.

Conclusion

The addition of healing beverages to your meals creates a tasty method to support your entire health system and general well-being. Every ingredient used in these beverages stays whole and final, which makes them transfer important nutrients while enabling your body's recovery through its natural healing pathways, resulting in an improved daily wellness outcome. A holistic approach highlights wholesome natural foods and drinks that contribute to sustainable health and lasting vitality.

33. The 30-Day Disease Prevention Routine

A full prevention strategy against diseases requires people to select their food carefully while maintaining their physical activity along with learning stress control and making meaningful changes to their way of life. A holistic approach emphasizes the importance of insightful health practices for immune strengthening, disease protection, and enhanced vitality. A thirty-day method has been created to set and strengthen enduring wellness practices.

Week 1: Establishing the Basics

A daily checklist for Days 1-7 emphasizes both proper nutrition and hydration, which includes the following components:

• Each morning, begin your day with a warm lemon water solution to enhance digestive health and purify the body.

• Unbalance your breakfast with protein combined with healthy fats as well as fiber by choosing foods such as avocado toast, smoothie bowls, and oatmeal.

• You should consume five parts from the vegetable and fruit groups in your daily meals.

• Drinking 8 cups of water per day should be your daily goal.

• Whole foods that lack processing and sugars should substitute processed items in people's diets.

• Selecting nutritious snacks includes portions of hummus and vegetable sticks along with nuts and fresh fruit as backup options.

Example Meal Plan:

• Breakfast: Greek yogurt parfait with berries and granola.

• Lunch: Quinoa and veggie salad.

- Dinner: Baked salmon with quinoa and steamed vegetables.

- The snack combination includes apple slices paired with almond butter.

Week 2: Enhancing Nutritional Intake

A daily checklist for Days 8-14 emphasizes both superfoods and nutrient-dense foods, which includes the following components

- Your eating plan should include superfoods, which comprise berries together with leafy greens, chia seeds, and nuts.

- One green smoothie daily should contain spinach together with banana and chia seeds.

- Healthy fats: Include sources like avocados, nuts, and olive oil.

- Your gut benefits from including yogurt together with kefir and sauerkraut, and kimchi to your daily food intake.

- Whole grains: Choose options like quinoa, brown rice, and oats.

Example Meal Plan:

- Breakfast: Berry and spinach smoothie bowl.

- Lunch: Mediterranean chickpea salad.

- Dinner: Chickpea and spinach curry with brown rice.

- Snack: Trail mix with nuts, seeds, and dried fruit.

Week 3: Building Physical and Mental Resilience

A daily checklist for Days 15-21 emphasizes both exercise and stress management, which includes the following components

- The exercise goal should be at least 30 minutes of moderate physical activities distributed across five days per week by performing activities like walking and jogging and practicing yoga.

- Two sessions of strength training should consist of bodyweight exercises and resistance bands.

- One should practice stretching through daily sessions of yoga or stretch exercises due to their impact on flexibility together with stress reduction benefits.

- Practice mindfulness and meditation techniques every day for a minimum of 10 to 15 minutes.

- To experience quality nocturnal rest you should attain between 7 to 9 hours of sleep in each 24-hour period.

Example Exercise Routine:

- Monday: 30-minute walk + 10 minutes stretching.

- Tuesday: Strength training + 15-minute meditation.

- Wednesday: 30-minute yoga session.

- Thursday: 30-minute jog + 10 minutes stretching.

- Friday: Strength training + 15-minute meditation.

- Saturday: 30-minute walk.

- Sunday: Rest day with light stretching.

Week 4: Solidifying Habits and Mindful Living

The daily checklist for incorporating holistic health practices runs from 22-30.

- The daily approach should include maintaining well-balanced dietary nutrition by eating whole foods over nutrient-rich meals.

- Maintain your regular routine of physical exercise which you have already established.

- You should practice mindfulness practices together with relaxation methods for daily use, such as deep breathing and gratitude journaling.

- Speaking with friends and family helps promote mental health stability.

- Make time for activities that generate pleasure and serve to relax you.

Example Daily Routine:

- Morning: Warm lemon water, healthy breakfast, and 10 minutes of mindfulness.

- Eating a balanced lunch should be combined with a half-hour exercise session or leisurely walk during midday.

- When the afternoon arrives, I usually consume a nutritious snack followed by stretching or practicing yoga.

- Evening: Nutritious dinner, quality time with loved ones, and a relaxing bedtime routine.

Herbal Supplements and Dietary Plan for Holistic Health

Recommended Herbal Supplements

- Echinacea: Boosts immune function (follow dosage instructions on the product).

- The consumption of turmeric provides anti-inflammatory benefits when using 1-2 teaspoons of ground turmeric in doses recommended by the package.

- In order to manage stress, Ashwagandha should be taken following the clear product instructions.

- Ginger helps digestion and minimizes inflammation through either fresh tea or supplement form.

Balanced Dietary Plan

- Breakfast: Energizing options like smoothies, oatmeal, or avocado toast.

- Lunch: Nutritious salads, grain bowls, or healthy wraps.
- Dinner: Protein-rich meals with vegetables and whole grains.
- Snacks: Fresh fruits, nuts, seeds, and yogurt.

Exercise and Mindfulness Activities Schedule for Holistic Health

Weekly Schedule

Monday:
- Morning: 30-minute walk
- Evening: 10-minute stretching

Tuesday:
- Morning: Strength training (bodyweight exercises)
- Evening: 15-minute meditation

Wednesday:
- Morning: 30-minute yoga session
- Evening: 10-minute mindfulness practice

Thursday:
- Morning: 30-minute jog
- Evening: 10-minute stretching

Friday:
- Morning: Strength training (resistance bands)
- Evening: 15-minute meditation

Saturday:
- Morning: 30-minute walk

- Evening: 10-minute relaxation exercise

Sunday:

- Morning: Rest day with light stretching
- Evening: 10-minute gratitude journaling

Conclusion

Through its 30-Day Disease Prevention Routine, professionals obtain a full system to build sustainable healthy habits. The combination of a nutritious diet with steady exercise, stress control, and a life with awareness will create strong support for your entire health system. A comprehensive approach highlights the importance of incorporating wellness practices into daily routines to support long-term health and disease prevention.

Appendix

1. Preparing Herbal Remedies

Natural remedies found in herbs strengthen both your health management and the support of medical conditions, as well as boost your general wellness. One should utilize premium natural elements when creating herbal medical treatments. The guide contains step-by-step instructions that cover the preparation of herbal tinctures and teas and also teach readers how to create salves while delivering essential storage information and utilization details.

Making Herbal Tinctures

Ingredients and Equipment:

- Fresh or dried herbs (e.g., echinacea, chamomile, valerian root)
- High-proof alcohol (e.g., vodka, brandy) or apple cider vinegar for a non-alcoholic tincture
- Glass jars with tight-fitting lids
- Cheesecloth or fine mesh strainer
- Different storage tools consist of dark glass bottles along with droppers as the receptacle.

Instructions:

1. **Prepare the Herbs:**

- Fresh herbs need rinsing before being reduced into small pieces.
- To create better contact between dried herbs, you must gently crush them before use.

2. **Fill the Jar:**

- The glass jar should receive about half of the herb material.

3. **Add the Solvent:**

- Add the apple cider vinegar or alcohol solvent to completely coat the herbs that fill the glass jar. The level of solvent should exceed the herbs by approximately 1 inch.

4. **Seal and Store:**

- Place an airtight seal on the jar, then store it inside a dark and cool area. Periodic daily shaking of the jar will optimize the extraction process.

5. **Strain the Tincture:**

- Carry out the extraction process by straining herbs through cheesecloth or a fine mesh strainer after allowing them to rest for 4-6 weeks while squeezing out all obtainable liquid.

6. **Bottle the Tincture:**

- Transfer the liquid to dropper-equipped dark glass bottles. Place the jar storage label with two pieces of information: the herb name and the tincture preparation date.

Usage:

- The required dosage of herbs depends on the specific herb together with the targeted medical condition. To use the herbal tincture take 1-2 droppers each time (one half to one full teaspoon) mixed with water or juice between two to three times during the day.

Brewing Herbal Teas

Ingredients and Equipment:

- Fresh or dried herbs (e.g., chamomile, peppermint, ginger)
- Teapot or heatproof glass jar

- Boiling water
- Tea strainer or infuser

Instructions:

1. Prepare the Herbs:

- Fresh herbs require rinsing, after which you must chop them before use.

- The proper measurement for dried herbs requires whole or crushed leaves and flowers or roots.

2. Measure the Herbs:

- Use about 1 tablespoon of fresh herbs or 1 teaspoon of dried herbs per cup of water.

3. Brew the Tea:

- Place the herbs in a teapot or jar. Jug the boiling water over the placed herbs before covering the pot. Let steep for 5-10 minutes.

4. Strain and Serve:

- A tea strainer or infuser will be used to separate the herb mixture from the water into the desired cup. You may enhance the beverage with honey or lemon to your taste.

Usage:

- Consumers should drink one to three cups per day according to herb and condition specifications.

Crafting Herbal Salves

Ingredients and Equipment:

- Dried herbs (e.g., calendula, comfrey, lavender)
- Olive oil or coconut oil
- Beeswax

- A pot of simmering water should support a double boiler or heatproof bowl for preparation.
- Cheesecloth or fine mesh strainer
- Small glass jars or tins for storage

Instructions:

1. **Infuse the Oil:**

- To prepare the oil infusion, you should place dried herbs inside a jar, followed by adding olive or coconut oil then secure the container. After placing the lid on the jar position it under direct sunlight for 2 to 4 weeks while daily shaking maintains the mixture.
- Heat the herbs with oil using a double boiler set at low temperature for a duration of 2 to 3 hours.

2. **Strain the Oil:**

- To extract the oil, you should use cheesecloth or a strainer with small holes while pressing down on the oil to drain it thoroughly.

3. **Prepare the Salve:**

- The strained oil should go into a double boiler for measurement purposes before pouring it into the device. You need one-fourth of a cup of beeswax for each cup of infused oil.
- Add heat to the mixture at a low temperature to melt the beeswax while occasionally stirring the mixture.

4. **Pour and Cool:**

- Put the mixture into multiple glass jars or tins before executing complete cooling that requires you to seal the containers.

Usage:

- Use the prepared salve to treat skin areas that need relief from irritation or dryness or minor wound treatment.

Storage and Usage Instructions for Herbal Remedies

Storage Tips:

•	Dark glass dropper bottles serve as proper storage for tinctures in a location that maintains both darkness and coolness. The correct storage methods allow tinctures to maintain their quality for several years.

•	Dried herb teas should be placed inside sealed airtight containers which should stay in a dark and cool environment. The product maintains its optimal effect if used within one year after preparation.

•	Salves must be stored inside small glass jars or tins in a dark and cool environment. Use within 6-12 months.

General Usage Guidelines:

•	The amount of tincture solution depends on both the herb type and the treatment requirement. People should take 1-2 dropper loads (equivalent to 1/2 to 1 teaspoon) of diluted liquid twice to three times each day.

•	Drink between one to three cups of herbal tea each day based on the type of herb along with the targeted medical condition.

•	The application of salves should be limited to required areas of the skin for managing skin irritations as well as dryness and minor wound recovery needs.

Safety Precautions:

•	A healthcare provider should guide decisions about new herbal treatments particularly when the patient is pregnant or nursing or taking medications.

•	Apply a small piece of the herbal product to your skin to check for allergic reactions after leaving it in place for twenty-four hours.

•	Select your herbal products from trustworthy vendors because they deliver more concentrated and medically safe compounds.

Conclusion

The home production of herbal treatments lets you access natural healing compounds that promote your overall health improvement. Following these practical instructions enables you to make herbal tinctures while also producing teas and salves that offer natural pain relief and general health benefits. Holistic method natural ingredients of high standard remain essential to produce the optimal effects from herbal medicine.

2. Comprehensive Shopping List for the Healing Kitchen

The fundamental aspect of a healing kitchen consists of assembling untainted, unprocessed foods that benefit wellness. One must incorporate nutrient-rich food components into their eating habits. The list encompasses everything needed for making healthy meals and beverages that support both short-term immunity strength and sustained overall well-being.

Fresh Produce

Fruits

- Apples
- Bananas
- Berries (blueberries, strawberries, raspberries, blackberries)
- Citrus fruits (lemons, oranges, grapefruits)
- Avocados
- Grapes
- Kiwis
- Mangoes
- Pineapples
- Melons (cantaloupe, watermelon)

- Pears

Vegetables

- Leafy greens (spinach, kale, Swiss chard, arugula)
- Cruciferous vegetables (broccoli, cauliflower, Brussels sprouts, cabbage)
- Root vegetables (carrots, sweet potatoes, beets, turnips)
- Squash (butternut, acorn, zucchini)
- Bell peppers
- Cucumbers
- Tomatoes
- Onions
- Garlic
- Celery
- Mushrooms
- Green beans
- Asparagus
- Leeks
- Radishes

Whole Grains and Legumes

- Quinoa
- Brown rice
- Wild rice
- Oats
- Barley

- Farro
- Lentils (green, red, black)
- Chickpeas (canned or dried)
- Black beans (canned or dried)
- Kidney beans (canned or dried)
- Navy beans (canned or dried)
- Split peas

Nuts, Seeds, and Healthy Fats

- Almonds
- Walnuts
- Cashews
- Pistachios
- Sunflower seeds
- Pumpkin seeds
- Chia seeds
- Flaxseeds
- Hemp seeds
- Nut butters (almond butter, peanut butter)
- Olive oil
- Coconut oil
- Avocado oil

Dairy and Dairy Alternatives

- Greek yogurt (plain, unsweetened)

- Kefir (plain, unsweetened)
- Almond milk (unsweetened)
- Coconut milk (unsweetened)
- Oat milk (unsweetened)

Herbs and Spices

- Fresh herbs (parsley, cilantro, basil, mint, rosemary, thyme, dill)
- Dried herbs (oregano, basil, thyme, rosemary, dill)
- Spices (turmeric, ginger, cinnamon, cumin, paprika, smoked paprika, chili powder, black pepper)
- Garlic powder
- Onion powder
- Sea salt or Himalayan salt

Sweeteners

- Honey
- Maple syrup
- Stevia (optional)

Baking Essentials

- Almond flour
- Coconut flour
- Whole wheat flour
- Baking soda
- Baking powder
- Vanilla extract
- Cocoa powder

Snacks

- Hummus
- Veggie sticks (carrots, celery, bell peppers)
- Whole grain crackers
- Rice cakes
- Dark chocolate (70% cacao or higher)
- Dried fruit (unsweetened, no added sugars)

Beverages

- Herbal teas (chamomile, peppermint, ginger, green tea, turmeric)
- Coconut water
- Lemon juice (fresh or bottled)

Condiments and Sauces

- Apple cider vinegar
- Balsamic vinegar
- Tamari or soy sauce (low sodium)
- Mustard (Dijon or whole grain)
- Tahini
- Salsa (no added sugars)
- Hot sauce (optional)

Frozen Foods

- Frozen berries (blueberries, strawberries, raspberries, blackberries)
- Frozen vegetables (spinach, broccoli, cauliflower, peas)
- Frozen fish (salmon, mackerel, cod)

- Frozen shrimp

Proteins

- Fresh fish (salmon, mackerel, cod)
- Poultry (chicken breasts, thighs, ground turkey)
- Lean meats (grass-fed beef, lamb)
- Tofu
- Tempeh
- Eggs

Superfoods

- Spirulina powder
- Matcha powder
- Goji berries
- Cacao nibs

Supplements (optional, based on individual needs)

- Echinacea tincture
- Turmeric capsules or powder
- Ashwagandha capsules or powder
- Ginger capsules or powder

Weekly Shopping Lists Aligned with the 30-Day Meal Plan

Week 1

- Fresh Produce: Spinach, avocados, bananas, berries, carrots, tomatoes, onions, garlic, lemons
- Whole Grains and Legumes: Quinoa, brown rice, chickpeas

- Nuts, Seeds, and Healthy Fats: Almonds, chia seeds, olive oil
- Dairy and Dairy Alternatives: Greek yogurt, almond milk
- Herbs and Spices: Fresh parsley, cilantro, turmeric, cumin, black pepper
- Snacks: Hummus, veggie sticks
- Beverages: Herbal teas (chamomile, peppermint), lemon juice

Week 2

- Fresh Produce: Kale, cucumbers, bell peppers, celery, apples, pears, grapes, ginger
- Whole Grains and Legumes: Lentils, oats, black beans
- Nuts, Seeds, and Healthy Fats: Walnuts, sunflower seeds, coconut oil
- Dairy and Dairy Alternatives: Kefir, coconut milk
- Herbs and Spices: Fresh mint, basil, cinnamon, garlic powder
- Snacks: Whole grain crackers, dark chocolate
- Beverages: Green tea, coconut water

Week 3

- Fresh Produce: Swiss chard, broccoli, sweet potatoes, mushrooms, avocados, pineapples, oranges
- Whole Grains and Legumes: Wild rice, navy beans
- Nuts, Seeds, and Healthy Fats: Cashews, pumpkin seeds, avocado oil
- Dairy and Dairy Alternatives: Oat milk
- Herbs and Spices: Fresh rosemary, thyme, paprika, onion powder
- Snacks: Rice cakes, dried fruit

- Beverages: Turmeric tea, matcha powder

Week 4

- The shopping list includes fresh produce such as arugula alongside cauliflower, as well as beets and, zucchini, and radishes together with melons and kiwis.

- Whole Grains and Legumes: Barley, kidney beans

- Nuts, Seeds, and Healthy Fats: Pistachios, hemp seeds, nut butter

- Dairy and Dairy Alternatives: Coconut milk

- The ingredients include fresh dill and oregano, together with smoked paprika and sea salt.

- Snacks: Salsa, hot sauce

- Beverages: Apple cider vinegar, balsamic vinegar.

Techniques for Preserving Nutrients in Foods

Storage Tips

- The refrigerator provides an optimal environment to store fresh produce because it protects both fresh content and nutritious value.

- You can protect food nutrients by freezing specific produce items that you will not use within a short period.

- Seal grains along with nuts inside tightly closed containers while placing them in dark, cool conditions for spoilage prevention.

Cooking Methods

- Steaming: Preserves the most nutrients in vegetables.

- Sautéing: Use a small amount of healthy fats like olive oil or coconut oil.

- The roasting method both boosts flavor and sustains nutritional content, especially if the temperature stays low during the process.

- The process involves quickly boiling vegetables before submerging them into ice water to retain their color along with texture and nutritional content.

Safe and Effective Detoxification Practices

- Your body needs at least 8 cups of water daily to support the removal of harmful substances from your system.

- Your body requires fiber-rich foods in large amounts because they help digestion and play a key role in detoxification processes.

- Your diet should include detoxing foods, which include garlic, beets, leafy greens and other similar vegetables.

- The natural detox process benefits from practicing intermittent fasting to provide periods where your digestive system has rest.

- Regular physical exercise enables sweating and helps eliminate toxins in your body.

Conversion Charts

Measurement Conversions

- 1 tablespoon = 3 teaspoons
- 1 cup = 16 tablespoons
- 1 ounce = 2 tablespoons (liquid)
- 1 ounce = 28 grams (dry)
- 1 pound = 16 ounces

Temperature Conversions

- 350°F = 175°C
- 400°F = 200°C
- 425°F = 220°C

Conclusion

Toward health and well-being everyone should maintain nutritious whole-food ingredients in their kitchen supplies. This entire shopping list, coupled with its foods, enables you to make healthy meals that benefit your long-term well-being. A holistic wellness system emphasizes the use of whole, natural ingredients that support the body's healing processes and maintain overall energy levels.

3. Techniques for Preserving Nutrients in Foods

Keeping food nutrients intact is essential because it sustains the health benefits of the food content. Maximizing the retention of essential vitamins, minerals, and other vital nutrients should be a priority in food preparation and processing to support overall health and well-being. The guide delivers methods to maintain nutritional value in your food desert to render kitchen recipes.

Storage Tips

Refrigeration

•   Fresh produce, including fruits and vegetables should stay in your refrigerator crisper drawer for better freshness and nutrient retention.

•   Fresh greens should receive protection by placing them in a plastic bag containing a dampened paper towel.

•   Herbs should be placed inside the refrigerator with their stems in water, forming a bouquet, and secured using a loosely placed plastic bag.

•   Dairy and Alternatives: Keep dairy products and plant-based alternatives in the coldest part of the refrigerator, usually the back.

Freezing

•   You should freeze extra fruits alongside vegetables since this method helps save their nutritional value. Freezing requires blanching vegetables immediately because it stops enzymes from decomposing flavors and affecting color while damaging texture.

- Fresh herbs require chopping before you store them in frozen ice tray cubes which need both water and olive oil. Freeze the herb cubes after they have reached their frozen state and put them inside a freezer bag.

- The freezer serves as an optimal storage solution for grains, nuts, along seeds since it protects their nutritional content and stops the development of rancidity.

Airtight Containers

- Store grains, as well as nuts and seeds, inside airtight containers within dark and cool areas for long-term preservation while protecting their nutritional value.

- You should use airtight containers to preserve dried fruits along with vegetables to protect their nutritional value while stopping the absorption of water.

Cooking Methods

Steaming

- When it comes to vegetable cooking, steaming stands as the method that best protects nutrients since it reduces losses when compared to alternative preparation methods. The method helps protect nutrients because it reduces both heat and water exposure.

- A steamer basket should cover boiling water to achieve this technique. Steam vegetables religiously until they reach the tender-crisp stage during 5-10 minutes of cooking time.

Sautéing

- Sautéing with a small amount of coconut oil or olive oil enables the retention of nutrients while also aiding fat-soluble vitamin (A, D, E, and K) absorption into the body.

- You should heat the oil to medium before adding vegetables until they become tender while staying vivid in color during this 5 to 10-minute cooking period.

Roasting

- The roasting process both enhances vegetable tastes and maintains nutritional content, especially when roasting occurs at reduced temperatures.

- The process involves spreading vegetables coated with a minimal amount of olive oil on a tray for roasting at 375°F (190°C) until they become tender for 20-30 minutes.

Blanching

- Using the blanching process, vegetables stay vibrant, and their textures and essential nutrients persist following boiling, followed by an ice bath.

- Place vegetables inside boiling water for 2-5 minutes to prepare them according to this technique. Quickly move the vegetables into ice water to prevent further cooking after they have been submerged.

Grilling

- The cooking method of grilling results in tasty dishes without requiring large quantities of fats, and it maintains vegetable nutrients during preparation.

- To grill the vegetables, consumers should preheat the grill first, then lightly brush them with olive oil before placing them over medium heat until they become tender for approximately 5-10 minutes on each side.

Microwaving

- Microwaving serves as a beneficial cooking method because it retains nutrients through brief cooking durations and small water usage.

- The microwave technique requires placing vegetables into a covered dish with small water amounts and setting the heat to high for 3-5 minutes until they become tender.

Minimizing Nutrient Loss

Reduce Water Use

- The cooking time should be short while maintaining minimal water levels because it halts the extraction of water-soluble vitamins B and C. Roasting and steaming and using the microwave produce excellent outcomes.

Shorten Cooking Time

- To maintain vegetable nutrients keep them in the cooking pot just until they reach tenderness. Excessive cooking eliminates essential vitamins C and various B vitamins from damaged food structures.

Use Cooking Water

- To maintain valuable nutrients in vegetables, you should use the discarded boiling water for creating soups, stews or sauces.

Avoid Peeling

- Always consume vegetables along with their skin since this outer portion retains plenty of nutrients in addition to dietary fiber.

Safe and Effective Detoxification Practices

Hydration

- A benefit of daily water consumption is that it removes waste products from the body alongside promoting wellness for the entire system.

- Drinking eight cups of water daily combined with consuming hydrating fruits and vegetables leads to improved health benefits.

Fiber-Rich Foods

•	The benefit of fiber intake involves its ability to remove toxins from our body and benefit digestion.

•	Your diet should contain many fruits, vegetables, whole grains, and legumes alongside other food items.

Detoxifying Foods

•	Specific foods implement natural detoxification processes in the body.

•	Examples: Garlic, beets, leafy greens, lemon, and turmeric.

Intermittent Fasting

•	The rest your digestive system receives through fasting helps your body conduct natural detoxification and enhances your metabolic well-being.

•	The 16/8 intermittent fasting technique (16 hours of fasting with 8 hours for eating) serves as a useful tip for detoxification.

Regular Exercise

•	The process of exercising causes sweating, that enables our bodies to eliminate toxins by releasing them through the skin.

•	You should perform moderate exercise for at least 30 minutes on most days throughout the week.

Conclusion

The process of retaining food nutrients requires storing them correctly, together with selecting suitable cooking methods and performing careful preparation techniques that prevent nutrient breakdown. Various nutritional methods enable you to obtain the maximum health value from your food while upholding your general wellness. A comprehensive approach that prioritizes nutrient retention in food supports long-term health benefits and overall well-being.

4. Safe and Effective Detoxification Practices

The body requires detoxification to eliminate dangerous substances, which supports general health. An organic approach to body purification combines effectiveness with safety, supporting overall well-being through natural methods. The guide presents actionable methods and techniques to clean the body through safe methods that preserve optimal health.

1. Hydration

Importance

- The intake of generous water amounts helps eliminate toxic matter and strengthens kidney function while maintaining proper hydration levels in the body.

Tips

- Every person should consume 8 cups of water throughout each day.

- Your water consumption becomes more appealing by adding lemon slices and cucumber along with mint because these items deliver both flavor enhancement and detoxifying advantages.

- You should prepare your herbal tea beverages from dandelion, ginger, and green tea because these plants support your body's detox process.

2. Fiber-Rich Foods

Importance

- The digestive system depends on dietary fiber to push toxins out because fiber also supports the health of the intestines.

Tips

- Fruits and Vegetables: Include a variety of fiber-rich fruits and vegetables such as apples, berries, carrots, and leafy greens.

- Whole Grains: Choose whole grains like quinoa, brown rice, oats, and barley.
- Legumes: Incorporate beans, lentils, and chickpeas into your diet.

3. Detoxifying Foods

Importance

- Liver detoxification receives support from natural foods that possess detoxifying qualities together with other detoxification processes.

Examples

- The sulfur compounds in garlic activate the liver enzymes to help remove toxins from the body.
- Beets provide the liver with multiple antioxidants along with nutritional elements that help the detoxification process.
- Leafy Greens contain chlorophyll which functions as a blood-purifying agent to promote liver health.
- The bile production promotion functions of lemon help both digestion and detoxifying processes.
- Turmeric contains curcumin, which benefits liver health while providing anti-inflammatory properties to the body.

4. Intermittent Fasting

Importance

- Your digestive system benefits when you practice intermittent fasting since this approach helps your body naturally detoxify itself.

Tips

- Through the 16/8 Method, you should fast for 16 hours but consume foods only during an 8-hour block. The eating window runs from midday at 12 PM until nighttime conclusion at 8 PM.

- You should eat a normal diet for five days before restricting your calories to 500-600 for any two separate days.

5. Regular Exercise

Importance

- Regular physical exercise produces sweating that enables the skin to remove toxins while benefiting your metabolic system.

Tips

- A routine of at least 30 minutes of moderate exercise should include walking, jogging, cycling, and swimming performed throughout most weekly days.

- Perform strength training exercises two or three times weekly because such workouts help build muscles while enhancing your metabolism.

- Practicing yoga brings two major benefits because yoga poses help with both flexibility and stress reduction, and specific yoga postures stimulate the lymphatic system for detoxification purposes.

6. Adequate Sleep

Importance

- Natural detoxification within the body depends heavily on sufficient sleep duration.

- The removal of brain toxins occurs as an essential part of natural brain detoxification through bodily processes.

Tips

- People need to establish a sleep pattern that maintains 7-9 hours of good sleep duration throughout each night.

- You should create a soothing evening routine, which might include reading, meditation, or bathing in warm water to help you sleep well.

- A properly set up sleep environment should include a delicate temperature with low light exposure.

7. Stress Management

Importance

- Long-lasting stress causes problems for your body when it tries to cleanse itself from harmful substances. A stress management plan promotes both human health and the detoxification process.

Tips

- Practice meditation along with deep breathing exercises and yoga since these mindfulness methods decrease stress.

- You should participate in activities that assist with relaxation, including outdoor time along with reading books, and music listening.

- Your emotional health benefits when you stay linked to family members along with your close friends.

8. Limit Exposure to Toxins

Importance

- Shortening your contact with environmental toxins allows your body to carry less toxicity load.

Tips

- Family life becomes healthier when you use natural cleaning substances instead of toxic chemicals.

- The purchase of organic foods should be your priority since this practice helps decrease exposure to pesticides and other chemicals.

- The consumption of filtered water protects you from chlorine, heavy metals, and other environmental pollutants.

- You should use natural personal care items, including shampoos, together with soaps and lotions because they do not contain dangerous chemicals.

9. Support Liver Health

Importance

- The liver functions as the main detoxifying organ in the human body. Liver health must remain strong in order to perform its detoxification process correctly.

Tips

- Liver-Supporting Foods: Include foods like garlic, onions, cruciferous vegetables, beets, and turmeric in your diet.

- Patients should use herbal supplements like milk thistle along with dandelion root and artichoke extract to help their liver function (weariness should happen with medical supervision first).

10. Dry Brushing

Importance

- Regular dry brushing promotes the work of the lymphatic system as it removes dangerous toxins from your body.

Tips

- Apply a natural bristle brush to perform gentle skin movements traveling toward your heart to achieve the desired effect. Begin your dry brushing with your feet and move in an upward direction.

- The dry brushing practice should be performed every day or multiple times per week during the morning before taking a shower.

Conclusion

People can safely detox through a complete system of hydration regulation together with high-fiber nutrition toxin-eliminating foods, intermittent fasting exercise, and rest periods while controlling stress together with environmental substance reduction, liver health promotion, and skin surface stimulation. Your routine practices, which include these techniques, help your body activate phytochemical processes for detoxification while preserving your total health and wellness. The use of sustainable natural detox techniques supports both long-lasting vitality and enhanced health.

5. Conversion Charts

Conversion charts positioned near the kitchen help bakers and cooks sustain accurate measurements for their food preparation activities. A holistic approach to cooking emphasizes the use of natural ingredients, precisely measured to preserve a meal's nutritional value. The essential conversion tools include volume measurements as well as weight measurements, temperature measurements and standard replacements for components in cooking.

Volume Conversions

Metric	Imperial	US Customary
1 milliliter (ml)	0.034 fluid ounces	0.202 teaspoons
5 milliliters (ml)	0.169 fluid ounces	1 teaspoon
15 milliliters (ml)	0.507 fluid ounces	1 tablespoon
30 milliliters (ml)	1.014 fluid ounces	2 tablespoons / 1/8 cup
60 milliliters (ml)	2.029 fluid ounces	4 tablespoons / 1/4 cup
120 milliliters (ml)	4.057 fluid ounces	1/2 cup
240 milliliters (ml)	8.115 fluid ounces	1 cup
1 liter (L)	33.814 fluid ounces	4.227 cups

Weight Conversions

Metric	Imperial	US Customary
1 gram (g)	0.035 ounces	0.0022 pounds
100 grams (g)	3.527 ounces	0.220 pounds
500 grams (g)	17.637 ounces	1.102 pounds
1 kilogram (kg)	35.274 ounces	2.204 pounds

Temperature Conversions

Celsius (°C)	Fahrenheit (°F)
0°C	32°F
10°C	50°F
20°C	68°F
25°C	77°F
30°C	86°F
40°C	104°F
50°C	122°F
60°C	140°F
70°C	158°F
80°C	176°F
90°C	194°F
100°C	212°F
180°C	356°F
200°C	392°F
220°C	428°F

Conversion Formula:

- From Celsius to Fahrenheit: °F=(°C×9/5)+32
- From Fahrenheit to Celsius: °C=(°F−32)×5/9

Common Ingredient Substitutions

Baking

If you don't have	Use this instead
1 cup all-purpose flour	1 cup whole wheat flour or 1 cup gluten-free flour blend
1 cup butter	1 cup coconut oil or 1 cup olive oil
1 cup sugar	3/4 cup honey or 3/4 cup maple syrup
1 egg	1 tablespoon chia seeds or flaxseeds + 3 tablespoons water (let sit for 5 minutes to gel)
1 cup buttermilk	1 cup milk + 1 tablespoon vinegar or lemon juice (let sit for 5 minutes)
1 teaspoon baking powder	1/4 teaspoon baking soda + 1/2 teaspoon cream of tartar

Cooking

If you don't have	Use this instead
1 cup chicken broth	1 cup vegetable broth or 1 cup water + 1 teaspoon soy sauce
1 cup heavy cream	1 cup coconut cream or 1 cup cashew cream
1 tablespoon cornstarch	2 tablespoons all-purpose flour or 1 tablespoon arrowroot powder
1 clove garlic	1/8 teaspoon garlic powder
1 onion	1/2 cup chopped leeks or shallots

Dry to Liquid Conversions for Herbs and Spices

Fresh Herbs	Dried Herbs
1 tablespoon fresh	1 teaspoon dried
3 tablespoons fresh	1 tablespoon dried

When working with dried herbs you should use less quantity because their concentrated strength surpasses fresh herbs by magnitude.

Conclusion

The conversion charts, together with ingredient substitutions, provide you with tools to follow recipes correctly in your cooking and baking efforts.

These guidelines support the creation of nutritious, delicious meals while aligning with a holistic approach to health and wellness. Tools available through these guidelines will help you create nutritious meals by adapting your recipes as well as swapping ingredients for wholesome results.

Conclusion

Empowering Your Health Journey

A person pursuing better health requires a complete system that combines proper nutrition with exercise routines alongside stress reduction techniques along complete practices. Through a focus on whole natural foods and mindful living, optimal health can be achieved and sustained with consistent, holistic practices. The guidance in this document will enable you to gain control over your health so you can achieve a vital and healthy lifestyle.

Key Takeaways

Holistic Nutrition

•	Dietary development should focus on consuming whole foods, including fresh vegetables with fruits, grains, and lean proteins alongside healthy fats. Natural foods with minimal processing and elimination of sugar additives should be avoided.

•	Water intake should remain high during the day as it promotes both health conditions and cleanses the system.

•	Every eating session needs to contain equal portions of proteins and carbohydrates together with fats, which sustain your energy levels and activate your body systems.

Healing Practices

•	Natural remedies based on herbal medicine should be used to both heal specific conditions and sustain overall health. You should regularly prepare herbal teas along with tinctures and create salves for your daily usage.

- Safe detox methods, including intermittent fasting hydration and the consumption of fiber-rich foods, along with regular physical exercise, will enable your body to eliminate toxins efficiently.

Lifestyle and Wellness

- Regular exercise, which should combine cardiovascular exercises and strength training, allows people to support both physical health and mood while enhancing their well-being.

- You should develop mindfulness skills along with stress management techniques because they help both your mental state and minimize stress damage to your physical system.

- Your body needs perfect rest and sufficient sleep to heal naturally which will promote global health.

Practical Tools

- Cultivate meal planning before food preparation since it enables you to have nutritious choices on hand for maintaining your nutritional goals.

- Conversion Charts and Substitutions provide recipe developers with tools to modify nutrients and maintain catering to dietary needs through ingredient changes.

Personalized Health

- Devote attention to the signals which your body relays to you.

- Your bodily signals should guide you to modify both your way of life and food selections.

- When in doubt about your health regimen you should ask healthcare professionals or herbalists and nutritionists for their expert advice. They will help you create plans that match your individual needs.

Final Thoughts

The process of becoming empowered requires making purpose-driven decisions based on awareness which benefits your complete health system. A whole-person strategy helps you establish a healthful way of life that provides equal nourishment to your physical body and mental and spiritual aspects. A comprehensive approach emphasizes natural, sustainable techniques to help individuals achieve optimal health and well-being.

The personal path to better health continues forever. Pay homage to your accomplishments while sustaining your dedication to achievements and maintaining a receptive attitude toward learning and adaptation. Your dedication, together with mindfulness, will enable you to achieve better health, thus leading to a vital and satisfying lifestyle. These guidelines will help you establish a healthier and happier life ahead. Take the voyage as you learn to lead your life successfully in every domain.

Printed in Dunstable, United Kingdom